The Soft Tissue Release Handbook

Reducing Pain and Improving Performance

Mary Sanderson and Jim Odell

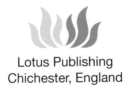

Lotus Publishing
Chichester, England

First published in 2012 by
Lotus Publishing,
Apple Tree Cottage, Inlands Road, Nutbourne, Chichester, West Sussex, PO18 8RJ, UK.

Anatomical Drawings Amanda Williams
Photographs Rufus Crosby
Text and Cover Design Wendy Craig
Printed and Bound in the UK by Scotprint

British Library Cataloguing-in-Publication Data
A CIP record for this book is available from the British Library
ISBN 978 1 905367 22 1

Contents

Introduction 7

Chapter 1: The Head and Neck 25
Chapter 2: The Shoulder Girdle Complex 45
Chapter 3: The Elbow 73
Chapter 4: The Forearm, Wrist and Hand 83
Chapter 5: The Torso: Thoracic and Lumbosacral Spine 95
Chapter 6: The Hip 117
Chapter 7: The Knee 137
Chapter 8: The Ankle and Foot 153

Case Studies 175
Resources 181
Index 187

Introduction

Soft tissue release (STR) is fast becoming a more and more popular massage technique, with practitioners from different spheres realising its benefits. This workbook has been inspired by many years of teaching and treating, with positive feedback from students in massage and clients on the plinth!

Case studies have shown that STR helps many common chronic conditions such as shoulder impingement, iliotibial band (ITB) friction syndrome and lateral epicondylitis. Experienced practitioners have found that skilled release of the soft tissues has reduced the need for adjustments or joint mobilisations because appropriate release improves joint movement. Freeing the joints and enhancing the health of the soft tissues also facilitate a superior and lasting response to rehabilitation programmes.

This book is aimed at anyone who wants to address the soft tissues precisely and effectively, whether as an adjunct to existing bodywork techniques or as a treatment modality in itself.

The book covers:

- Descriptions of normal movements in specific areas of the body

- Discussions of problems caused by soft tissue restrictions in these areas

- Demonstrations of how STR can be used to restore pain-free normal movement

The Role of Soft Tissue in Movement Restrictions and Pain

The soft tissues consist of muscle fibres, myofascia, tendons and ligaments. Each muscle fibre, each bundle of muscle fibres (or 'fascicule') and each muscle belly is encased in fascia, known as the endomysium, the perimysium and the epimysium respectively. This myofascia extends from the muscle to form the tendon, which melds into the periosteum of the bone to form a strong attachment.

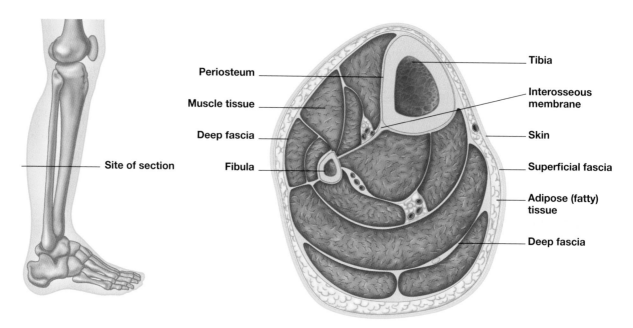

Figure 1: Cross section of skeletal muscle.

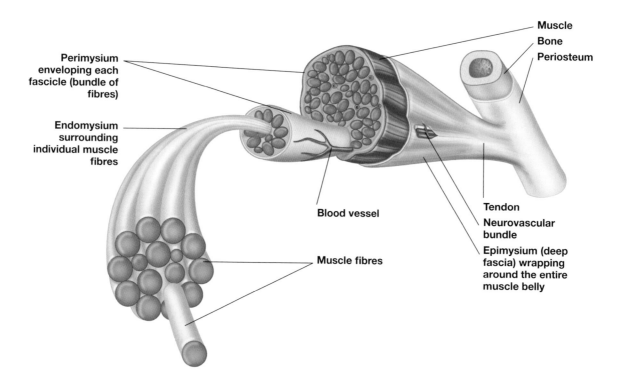

Figure 2: Layering of muscle and fascia.

Experienced body workers become fascinated with the all-encompassing nature of the fascia, this enveloping and supportive tissue where chronic injury resides. As our knowledge of the soft tissues increases, it becomes more apparent how inappropriate it is to try to separate out specific soft tissue structures and how essential it is to look at them as different forms of connective tissue with muscles embedded in them. Treatment of the soft tissues continues to gain momentum, and there are many exciting and interesting research developments that demonstrate how skilled manipulation of these tissues can have profound effects on the structure and function of the musculoskeletal system.

The Mechanism of Soft Tissue Injury

Within 20 minutes following a tissue tear, the repair process is initiated with inflammation. Muscle injury can be 'shearing', in which the connective tissue framework as well as the myofibres is torn, or it can be an in situ injury, where only the myofibres are torn. Inflammation is a positive and necessary phase which first protects the healing wound from infection and then starts the repair process. During the repair process the 'gluing' together is initiated: a blood clot and local cells bind to each other, and collagen fibres are laid down in a criss-cross mesh over the reticular fibres. However, this adhesion is not very strong and can easily be re-torn.

As the inflammation settles, after about two days (depending on the severity of the tear), fibroblastic activity commences. The migrating fibroblasts produce the collagen fibres, which are laid down along the lines of stress to bind and repair the wound; new capillaries, essential for getting oxygen to the regenerating tissue, are also formed from the undamaged vessels. Regeneration of intramuscular nerves also occurs. Neuromuscular junctions are resistant structures and the repairing axons join on to them. As collagen is made, so it is broken down as the remodelling process allows for the maturation of the regenerated tissue and contraction and re-absorption of the scarring. In muscle tissue it is the satellite cells that become activated by the necrosis of the myofibres, which proliferate and form into myotubes that then develop into myofibres. A balance between regeneration of new tissue and formation of scar tissue is necessary for optimal healing.

Tears in ligamentous tissue are referred to as 'sprains', whereas tears in muscle tissue are referred to as 'strains', 'contusions' or 'lacerations'. Practitioners often grade them according to the degree of damage and how many fibres seem to have been torn. Complete rupture will need surgical repair. Shearing muscle injuries result in severe bleeding: an intramuscular haematoma is where the bleeding is contained within the myofascia; an intermuscular haematoma is where the myofascia is torn and the blood spreads.

In most soft tissue injuries many different types of fibre are torn and in all cases their early mobility is essential.

Effect of Immobilisation

An initial period of immobilisation is necessary to allow for the formation of granular tissue; the length of time will depend on the grade of injury, but immobilisation should be kept to a minimum, as early mobility will keep the scar mobile. As the repair process gets under way it is necessary to move the fibres to encourage collagen to align along the lines of stress, to keep the connective tissue fibres lubricated and to encourage recapillarisation.

If active recovery is not followed, tissue strength and function will be compromised: since collagen is laid down randomly, there will be a decrease in tissue mobility where cross-links are formed in the collagen. Muscle tissue will tend towards shortening, with less sarcomeres and a thickening of its connective tissues; shortened muscle will reduce the range of motion (ROM) at the joint it crosses. Tendons will atrophy and the connective tissue of the tendon and its sheath will thicken and impede gliding; the tendon will have reduced strength for transferring the forces of the contracting muscle, and an inflammatory state can ensue. Ligaments will become lax and have impaired function in stabilising a joint during movement.

Connective tissues thicken and harden with injury. This prevents muscle fibres from moving efficiently and impairs their function. Rigid connective tissue also affects nervous, lymphatic and venous tissue pathways: this will influence the neural control of muscle tissue as well as the immune and circulatory functions of the body. Restriction and adhesion can occur in both superficial and deep fascia. In the deep fascia it can occur within a muscle, at the musculotendinous junction, within tendon sheaths, at the periosteum, between muscle bellies and between borders of muscles.

In addition to the above changes, many studies have shown that immobilisation also produces rapid reductions in muscle mass and strength, as well as negative changes in the structure of cartilage and bone, which can affect healing and store up problems for the future.

Shortened Muscle Tissue Reduces ROM of Joints

Many movement restrictions are a direct result of muscle shortening, primarily because of thickened myofascia. Muscle tissue is well vascularised and heals well. Cellular debris is cleared quickly in the inflammatory stage, and muscle regeneration can be completed three weeks after initial injury. It is restriction in the connective tissues and the reduced number of sarcomeres which impede a muscle's ability to maintain length.

It is necessary to lengthen shortened muscle tissue and enhance its health by tissue manipulation, but consideration of the coordination and strength of associated muscles is essential in maintaining improved and pain-free movement. Problems with the soft tissues will lead to changes in joint movement, and changes in joint movement will lead to injury in the soft tissues; it is not always easy to ascertain which happened first.

Strengthening of Inhibited Muscles

During immobilisation, muscles can become weak because of reduced activity. There may be obvious wastage – some muscles, such as the quadriceps, wasting faster than others – and progressive exercises are required to regain full strength and motor control.

With an overuse injury, in which pain and faulty movement patterns have developed gradually over a period of time, the strengthening of inhibited muscles needs to be considered more carefully. Skilled exercise prescription is essential in gaining full function; there are many methods of instruction, such as Pilates and the Feldenkrais Method, which are aimed at strengthening specific muscles while emphasising correct movement and control. Conditioning should be progressive.

Release of congested tissue prior to and in conjunction with strengthening programmes is vital in returning tissues to their pre-injured state and maximising their function. Actually engaging inhibited muscles will be easier if associated tight tissue has been released. For example, it would be very difficult to target 'core' abdominal muscles correctly, at the necessary subtle level, if layers of back muscles were tight and the fascial tissues sticky; the proprioception would be impaired, so the desired exercises are unlikely to be performed correctly. The only case in which it may be inappropriate to release the soft tissues prior to strengthening is an acute injury where an associated protective muscle spasm is in place; in this situation, rest and progressive mobility prior to muscle release and strengthening are recommended.

Many tendinopathies consist of weak and chronically inflamed structures. Resting from the initiating action, applying ice and performing appropriate strengthening exercises are prerequisite for repair. In the absence of tissue release, however, full function may never be recovered. It is necessary to release tissue congestion and ensure that the tendon sheaths are free from restrictions by treating the muscle, and the myofascia from which the tendon originates, to maximise conditioning effects. Body-wide influences of tissue congestion, muscle balance, strength and ROM are inevitably part of the treatment process.

The Overuse Injury (Repetitive Strain)

Tears to the soft tissues can occur at the microscopic level and go unnoticed, but the same mechanisms of tissue response through to regeneration and remodelling will still take place. The same impairments to full recovery, therefore, are still possible: a microscopic wound heals but the scar may not be completely reabsorbed, leaving the regenerated tissue slightly weaker and less mobile, which affects the overall function of the muscle and its synergists and antagonists.

Subtle changes in function in a local area over a period of time will affect a larger area. Sticking of muscle borders, shortened muscle groups, inhibited muscle groups, dehydrated rigid fascia – all of these factors increase the chance of a traumatic injury.

Physical exercise, mobility and stretching are essential for good health, and it is necessary to micro-traumatise muscle fibres in order for them to repair and strengthen: this is the training effect. Balanced training and recovery ensure that muscle tissue is regenerated, capillarisation is increased and neuromuscular pathways specific to the particular sport or activity are created. The repetitive nature of training for a sport, however, means that pain from overuse can develop. Whether it is clocking up the distance in running, swimming and cycling, or pumping iron in the gym, or persistently hitting a tennis ball with a racquet, the repetitive nature means that tearing in the soft tissues will inevitably occur and go unnoticed until a more serious pain or condition develops. Athletes are often unaware that they are not functioning to their full potential, because of a local tissue change that began months or even years previously. It may be that stride length has reduced, the foot is not being planted as efficiently or the spine has become less mobile. These factors not only impair function but may also increase an athlete's susceptibility to injury.

Furthermore, injuries which seem to be a result of sport are, in actual fact, largely due to everyday activities. Stiffness from a repetitive day-to-day activity can be the root cause of an injury which presented during vigorous activity. Many occupations, for example office work and driving, involve repetitive yet static positions. Sitting behind a computer for long periods will encourage the head and shoulder to protract forwards, particularly on the side that is manipulating the mouse. Dynamic jobs, for example the building trades, have their own set of issues, such as heavy lifting, repetitive bending and ladder work. These tasks can be made worse by unbalanced positions such as when carrying awkward loads. Compensation occurs, ultimately leading to an imbalance of musculature around a joint. General postural habits in daily life – such as slouching in a chair, twisting to view a television screen or favouring one leg in standing – must also be considered.

In all cases of overuse injury, unravelling the initial 'cause' of someone's pain can be complex and multifactorial. Rather than just addressing someone's symptoms, it is necessary to locate the cause of tissue dysfunction and provide advice on stretching and strengthening, for instance; often it may mean collaboration with trainers or coaches, or consideration of occupational positions.

Equipment	Activity	Rest	Biomechanics	Past influences
• Check equipment used in activity, e.g. weight, leverage and grip of a racquet • Correct set-up, e.g. bike • Footwear • Surface: court, road, track, terrain • Protective clothing • Office and home: position of chair, screen, mouse • Car seat • Sleeping: bed, pillows	• Sport-specific warm-up • Correct training: conditioning and technical aspects for the sport • Fitness: fatigue will affect resilience and ability to perform the correct technique • Check influences of day-to-day activities, such as correct lifting, bending, standing and sitting	• Appropriate cool-down • Recovery between training sessions • Recovery from repetitive actions or static positions in work or day-to-day activities • Good nutrition	• Relative strength between certain muscles • Flexibility specific to the activity • Posture • Core strength	• Previous injury • Congenital conditions, such as scoliosis and leg-length discrepancies • Age

Table 1: Considerations in the prevention of overuse injury.

Conditions That Affect Each Area of the Body

Assessment of the soft tissues can be done through palpation and analysing the movement pattern of a joint; with STR these can be done simultaneously. A particular reduction in an expected ROM is indicative of restrictions in certain muscle groups. When presented with a particular 'condition', however, it can be easy to suspect particular muscle groups and get drawn in to a certain routine. For example, two individuals may present with similar faulty movement of the scapula, but the therapist then finds that the soft tissues feel very different. It is essential to look beyond what seems to be the obvious problem, and treat according to what is felt under the hands. Checking ROM and assessing the texture of the soft tissues should be reconsidered, since these characteristics are unique for each individual.

'Feel' is an inexact science, and skilled palpation of the soft tissues only comes with years of experience and patient feedback; good listening and communication skills are essential for gauging sensation and levels of discomfort. When palpating the tissues it is important to understand the mechanism or injury that leads to these common soft tissue dysfunctions. Particular conditions in the soft tissues rarely occur in isolation and can vary hugely. The following background of common dysfunctions is used as a guide for developing touch skills.

Inflammation is the initial response to tissue trauma. It will present with one or more of the following symptoms: redness, swelling, pain and reduced ROM. Direct pressure to inflamed areas will cause further tissue damage. Rest, ice, compression and elevation (RICE) are recommended as initial treatment following any tissue trauma. Often treatment away from the inflammation is indicated to maintain good circulation, but it would be detrimental to provide any movement directly to the inflamed area. Commonly, chronic conditions – such as lateral epicondylitis or supraspinatus tendonitis – present with an area of inflammation. Avoid working directly on any acute tissue response, but STR can be performed very close to an inflamed area and have a positive impact on tissue repair without adversely affecting the inflammation.

Scar tissue is formed as a result of the repair process. Although initially it binds a wound, it is weaker than the tissue it has repaired: it lacks extensibility, strength and mobility. It can also feel hard and dense. Thorough rehabilitation will promote a complete recovery from any scarring and encourage regeneration of torn tissue. A heavier bleed with a larger number of torn fibres will lead to higher fibroblastic activity and, ultimately, more scar tissue formation. Pressure and movement are essential for a full recovery.

Adhesive tissue is where two structures that should be separate are sticking together. It can occur between any two gliding surfaces, such as muscle groups (e.g. the gastrocnemius and the soleus), between fasciculi, between tendons and their sheaths, between muscles and tendons (e.g. the vastus lateralis and the ITB), and in a capsular fold. As a result of tearing and an impaired gliding of the fibres, as well as a reduced lubrication of collagen fibres, extra cross-bridges can be laid down in the collagen matrix, and a thickening and gluing of connective tissues occurs. Locking into the tissues between adhering surfaces and lengthening the fibres facilitates separation.

Hypertonic muscle tissue is where there is too much tone in a muscle. Tight muscle will have increased tone and a decrease in its overall resting length. A muscle can also have increased tone without being shortened; in this case it could be said to be locked long.

Inhibited muscle is where there is a decrease in the muscle's strength. It may be that the muscle fibres cannot fire at their full potential because of altered biomechanics, or that a muscle has atrophied following injury. STR to opposing tight muscle groups will help in the specific strengthening of inhibited muscles.

Compartment syndrome is where a muscle or group of muscles within a fascial sheath (compartment) becomes swollen to the extent that there is a pressure build-up within the compartment. The pressure can cause compression of nerves and vascular structures. Acute compartment syndrome, often resulting from a direct blow, needs hospital attention. Chronic compartment syndrome, from overuse, is more likely to occur where the fascial sac is denser, such as in the anterior compartment of the lower leg; skilled use of STR can alleviate symptoms. The area may feel hard and sensitive.

STR and Adverse Neural Tension

Adverse neurological tension is any injury to the nervous system that in turn influences the function of the tissues elsewhere. This could involve changes to nerve impulses, blood supply, muscle strength or tone. The nervous system is commonly injured in the following locations:

- Soft tissue and/or bony tunnels – for example the median nerve in the carpal tunnel, or the tibial nerve in the tarsal tunnel.

- Where the nervous system is fixed – for example the peroneal nerve to the head of the fibula.

- Where the nervous system branches – for example where the branches of the lateral and medial nerves join to form the common plantar digital nerve between the third and fourth toes.

- Where the nervous system passes close to a structure that does not move – for example the brachial plexus as it goes over the first rib.

- At tension points – for example at the sixth thoracic vertebral level.

STR needs to be administered with care. Skilled use will release muscle compression on a nerve, such as in 'piriformis syndrome', but too much pressure which reproduces symptoms can be detrimental to healing. Since the STR lock is only momentary, harmful effects should not occur with skilled use.

STR Following Surgery

Following surgery and enforced immobilisation, adverse tissue changes will be more severe. The surgeon's blade causes laceration, which has to heal, and the subsequent enforced immobilisation means that tissues will thicken and adhere, and scarring will manifest. Muscle shortening and atrophy will be present, along with thickening and dehydration of fascial tissues.

	Healthy tissue texture	Unhealthy tissue texture
Muscle	Flexible, supple and pliant	Dense, cannot apply deep pressure, difficult to pick up, can feel flaccid if inhibited/wasted
Superficial fascia	A bow wave can be produced, moves easily in different directions	Feels clammy, difficult to move over underlying tissues
Myofascia	Easy to locate muscle borders and feel the outline of a muscle	Difficult to locate muscle borders, dense, 'thickened'
Tendon	Easy to grasp, firm	Thick, stringy, swollen
Ligament	Stiff	Lax and thin

Table 2: Summary of tissue texture.

Movement and Pressure Are Essential for Optimal Repair

Movement is essential for regeneration of damaged tissue and to loosen stiff and sticking tissue; manual pressure is also needed to release tissue restriction. The combination of pressure and movement is a powerful tool for any physical therapist. Adding in a functional component during STR and skilled muscle strengthening is a quick way of restoring strength, correct movement and coordination.

The Role of STR

STR is dynamic and participative and facilitates a fast relief of common soft tissue dysfunctions such as hypertonicity, scar tissue adhesions and lesions. It provides swift and lasting improvements to many chronic pain patterns and is perfect to use alongside other physical therapy techniques such as chiropractic, osteopathy and physiotherapy. Gentle STR can be used in the sub-acute phase of healing in conjunction with early mobility work, but its primary role is addressing chronic tissue changes.

STR is widely used in sporting circles, where it can be beneficial for sports people at any level:

• *Maintenance*

First, regular treatment can help maintain the physical form, speed up recovery from training and minimise the risk of injury. Treatment can identify early signs of soft tissue dysfunction and address it, thus ensuring that 'problem' areas do not go unnoticed. Keeping muscles and their supporting tissues pliant and in good health helps them to tolerate the rigours of training and minimises the risks of overuse injury.

- *Treatment of injury*

Second, in the event of an injury, STR is an effective tool to use in conjunction with rehabilitation. Problem areas can be located quickly and addressed accordingly. Because STR requires movement of the problem area, it involves the nervous system and facilitates the re-education of injured tissue.

- *Versatility*

Finally, it is a highly versatile technique, which can be advantageous at sporting events. In these situations there may be many variable parameters such as timing (when the athlete is due to compete) and facilities; STR is highly adaptable and can be performed through clothes or in a functional position as necessary.

STR is also a very useful soft tissue technique for reducing pain caused by day-to-day activities:

- *Physical jobs*

Physical jobs as well as sport can lead to injury. Regular STR will help identify early signs of tissue stress and can be an effective way of addressing problems while taking account of a person's occupation and its unique positions and movement patterns.

- *Static positions*

STR is a good way of bringing in movement in the case where static positions, such as when driving, are the cause of pain. It is an ideal technique for teaching someone to go through a range of motion and for encouraging self-treatment programmes.

- *Prevention*

Employers are becoming more aware of the need to prevent injury, both to reduce absenteeism through injury and to improve staff morale. Some offices even operate on-site massage schemes; STR is an ideal technique as it can be done quickly, without oils and with minimal disturbance.

How to Perform STR: 'Lock – Lengthen – Release'

To perform STR effectively it is vital to have a thorough knowledge of anatomy and good palpation skills; it is equally important to understand movement, acceptable variations and altered movement patterns that are indicative of pain and dysfunction.

Actually doing STR, however, is an ideal way of enhancing palpation skills and of gaining knowledge of anatomy, through touch and movement. Feeling fibres moving while treating them helps to locate attachments, separate borders and pinpoint more easily specific structures and particular tissue conditions.

The Technique

STR is performed by locking into the tissues and maintaining the lock while the aligning fibres are lengthened: lock – lengthen – release. The lock can be administered in many different ways, depending on what needs releasing and where. The lengthening, or stretch, can also vary.

The Lock

How the lock is administered will determine how effectively the soft tissues are released. There are many different ways of addressing the tissues, depending on their condition. The lock can be used to lengthen shortened muscle fibres. It can be used to separate adhesions between muscle groups or bellies within a muscle. Scar tissue can be locked into with a direct lock. Tendons can be isolated and the connective tissue matrix can be specifically targeted using a connective tissue massage (CTM) lock.

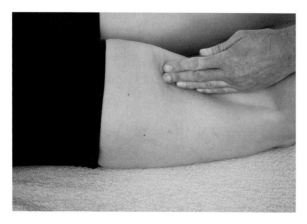
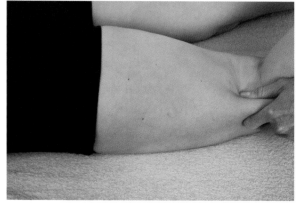

Depending on what needs to be done, the type of lock should take into account the following:

• **Surface area**: when first locking into the tissues, always start with a broader contact surface area.

• **Amount of pressure**: do not apply too much pressure too soon. If the tissue resists or tenses, the pressure should be reduced.

• **Direction of pressure**: think about how the tissues should feel. If the tendon fibres are bunched up and stringy, a broadening lock may be necessary. If a muscle is short, consider a lengthening lock away from the joint that is being moved, to enhance the stretch.

• **A CTM lock**: this is specifically designed to address the connective tissues. Areas where myofascia is particularly abundant – such as in the tibialis anterior, the infraspinatus, the thoracolumbar fascia and the plantar fascia – will benefit from a CTM lock. Any tendon can be treated with a CTM lock. Any location where the connective tissues feel thickened or tacked down will experience a faster and more lasting release if the tissue is addressed specifically with a CTM lock.

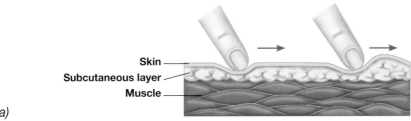

a)

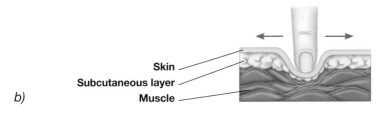

b)

Figure 3: A connective tissue massage (CTM) lock; a) superficial fascia, b) myofascial mobilisation into fascial layer of muscle.

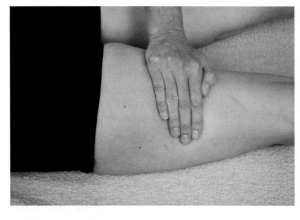
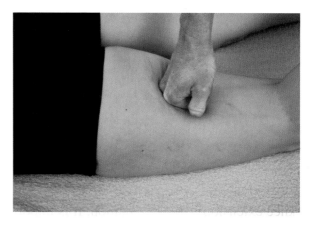

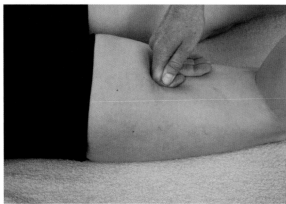
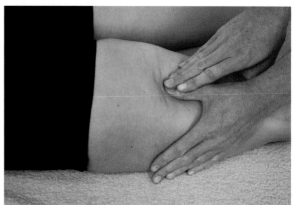

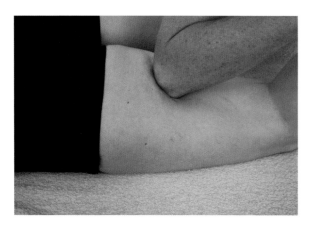

The hands and forearms are a therapist's tools, and they must be used intelligently with good body mechanics to maximise their efficiency; obviously, the therapist should also be aware of the need to reduce the risk of personal injury. Initially, where the tissues need to be softened and warmed up, a broad surface lock is recommended: the pressure is more superficial and over a broader area. Examples are: the whole hand, gently cupped, the heel of the hand, a broad surface ulna and a soft fist. For a deeper and more specific lock, fingers, thumbs or knuckles and elbows (olecranon) can be used. It is important to protect the hands to prevent injury to them. Ensure that a good working posture is adopted and that a correctly positioned couch at the right height is employed. Use body weight to gain pressure into the tissues. Always reinforce a lock where possible: for example, if using a thumb, reinforce it with the fingers of the other hand. There are massage tools available which can be helpful, but these should be used with care, as they will not have the same tissue feedback as the hands and forearms.

The Stretch

Movement in the form of lengthening can be administered passively by the therapist or actively by the subject; it can be minimal, to provide a very specific release, or it can be initiated through a fuller range. In congested and shortened areas it may be necessary to shorten the muscle first, prior to locking in and stretching.

When the muscle has more than one action, combinations of movements can occur. For example, when treating the hamstrings in the prone position, the tendons of insertion will benefit from knee extension and knee rotation. It is important to check the ROM before initiating any active stretch. Consider the joint selection when the muscle passes over more than one joint. In the case of the hamstrings, when working in the supine position, it may suit to flex the hip and extend the knee. It is advised to perform only one movement at a time to avoid tissue trauma.

The stretch should generally be performed slowly so that tissue responses can be felt and released after the required length has been attained. The lock is also released at this time. STR can be combined quite easily with muscle energy techniques (METs) such as active isolated stretching and 'hold-relax' techniques.

Different Types of STR

Passive STR is when the therapist locks into the tissues and manipulates the limb to produce the stretch. It is often done as a warm-up. Passive STR would be useful in the early stages of repair, in which case the lock would need to be gentle and the stretch performed within a pain-free ROM so as not to break the fragile granulation. It is also useful where movement is difficult for the subject, for example in cases of spasticity following a stroke or if there is severe muscle wastage.

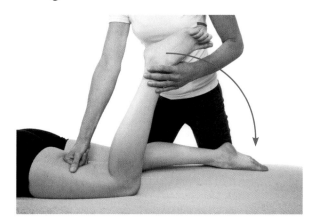 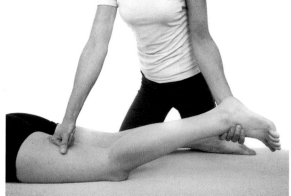

Active STR is when the therapist locks into the tissues and guides the subject into the appropriate movement to lengthen the fibres. This is less labour intensive for the therapist; it also empowers the subject. If any area is particularly congested, the subject can gain control when a release may be a little painful: the subject need only move as far as is comfortable.

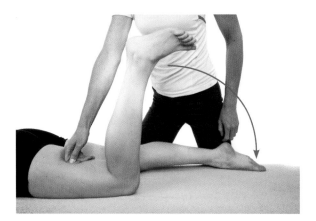 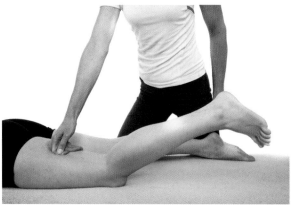

It is also a very useful way of teaching a subject to perform correctly a movement pattern that may not have been recognised as impaired or faulty, thus promoting functional awareness. Actively engaging the subject during treatment increases proprioception from the muscle spindles, stretch receptors and fascial proprioceptors. Involving the nervous system is a necessary part of any rehabilitation, and active STR combines this need for movement with manual pressure.

Weight-bearing STR is when the subject is in a functional position, for example standing. The therapist locks in and asks the subject to move into a stretch, or the subject holds something (such as a ball) and mimics a throwing action. This method can prove very useful for fine-tuning a particular movement pattern, and it is an invaluable part of rehabilitation. Sports people are often very specific about where their pain appears in a movement cycle, and this technique can be interactive with instant feedback.

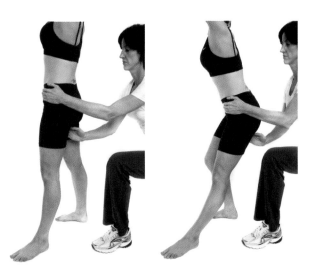

Resisted STR is when the therapist locks into the tissues but resists the subject's active stretch. It is a variation of active STR where it may be beneficial to control segmental movement by restraining the subject's movement. It also allows the tissues that are being worked on to relax through reciprocal inhibition (RI). This can be useful when it is difficult to achieve the desired depth because of severe tissue 'stickiness'.

Considerations

There are many things to take into account when administering STR to obtain maximum enhancement of the tissues. These considerations will vary from person to person and depend on the situation. For example, are you working at an event on a finely tuned athlete who has already warmed up? Or are you treating someone fresh out of a plaster of Paris cast, whose muscles and supporting connective tissues have not moved fully for a while? Factors to consider include:

- **Speed of application**: although STR is a dynamic technique, it is essential not to work too fast. Always allow time to 'feel' the tissues and how they are responding. Lock slowly to avoid crushing the tissues and to minimise tissue trauma.

- **Treatment of layers**: always treat superficial layers of tissue first.

- **Direction of movement**: when the lock is applied, it is often angled away from the joint that is being moved to lengthen the muscle fibres. In relation to the fascia, myofascia practitioners move along a fascial plane in the direction that the fascia needs to go; consider this when applying a CTM lock.

- **Breathing pattern**: follow the subject's breathing and give guidance when necessary. When applying a deeper lock, gain depth on the exhalation to help the subject maintain relaxation. In some cases it may take two or three exhalations as the pressure is increased to attain the required depth.

- **Movement selection**: passively guiding the subject through a stretch prior to active STR will ensure that the movement is performed correctly. Empower the subject to move within a comfortable range and guide an active stretch to re-educate where necessary. Consider joint movement selection if a muscle acts over more than one joint or if a muscle has more than one action.

- **Palpation tool**: use the dynamism of STR to assist with palpation. Feel the direction and depth of muscle fibres and how the tendons move.

- **Overview**: think beyond the tissue that is being treated. If nothing seems to be responding, move on. No two 'tennis elbows' will be the same: consider the common extensor tendon of the forearm and the extensor muscles, but also the triceps, the shoulder complex generally and the neck.

- **Timing**: be sympathetic to when the treatment is taking place in relation to sport training and competition, as well as in relation to work or day-to-day activities. For example, avoid significant release prior to a major competition, and consider how the particular release may affect performance. STR can affect performance at work or on a long journey, e.g. the client may feel tired or "spaced out" after treatment.

- **Unusual responses**: autonomic responses can occur particularly when treating extremely chronic conditions. These may take the form of nausea, body temperature change and tiredness. Should any of these occur, take a moment's break from treatment to allow the nervous system to settle.

The Head and Neck

1

Although there are many muscles located on and within the head and neck, the scope of this book will be confined to those soft tissue structures that are known to become tight or restricted or can be implicated in conditions that cause discomfort through dysfunctional movement and can be treated with STR. These will include muscles and other soft tissue associated with the temporomandibular joint and the joints of the cervical spine.

Head

Temporomandibular Joint (TMJ)

The TMJ is the articulation between the condyle of the mandible and the temporal bone. There is a fibrous, saddle-shaped meniscus separating the condyle and the temporal bone: it is attached to posterior soft tissues that allow the condyle to move forwards.

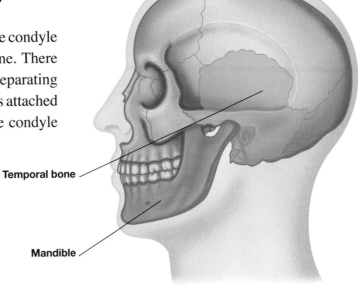

Temporal bone

Mandible

Figure 1.1: The TMJ and the skull.

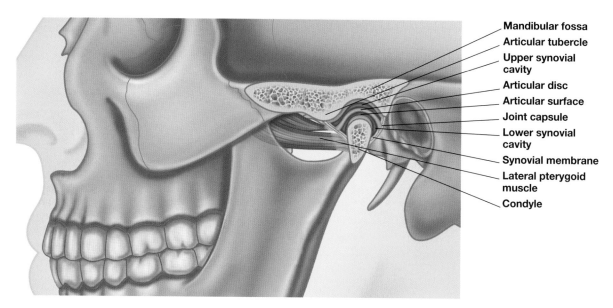

Mandibular fossa
Articular tubercle
Upper synovial cavity
Articular disc
Articular surface
Joint capsule
Lower synovial cavity
Synovial membrane
Lateral pterygoid muscle
Condyle

Figure 1.2: The TMJ.

Movement of the TMJ

Two key motions occur at the joint when the mouth opens. The first is rotation around an axis that passes through the condylar heads. The second is translation in which the condyle and meniscus both move anteriorly beneath the articular eminence. Mastication requires a more complex movement of the mandible involving depression with protrusion, lateral deviation, elevation with retrusion and medial deviation back to the start position.

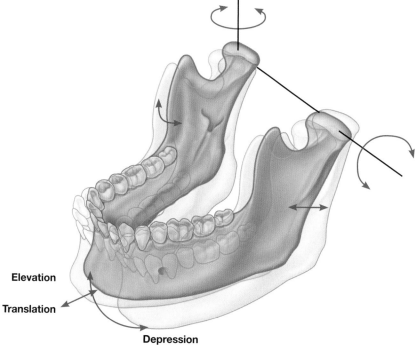

Elevation

Translation

Depression

Figure 1.3: TMJ movement.

Muscles of the TMJ

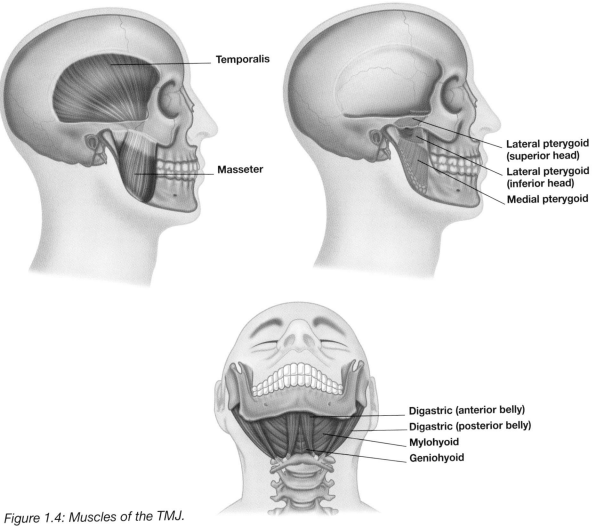

Figure 1.4: Muscles of the TMJ.

Muscle	Movement of the mandible				
	Depression	Lateral deviation	Elevation	Protrusion	Retrusion
Masseter		Ipsilateral	■		
Temporalis		Ipsilateral	■		■
Lateral pterygoid		Contralateral		■	
Medial pterygoid		Contralateral	■		
Mylohyoid	■				
Diagastric	■				
Geniohyoid	■				

Key	Primary role	Secondary role	Possible role

Table 1.1: Muscle movement at the TMJ.

Muscle	Effect of tightness
Masseter	Restricted jaw depression, lateral deviation of mandible (unilateral) with impact on bite mechanics. Compression of disc and tissue.
Temporalis	Similar to those of masseter but with greater effect. Static retraction of jaw and concomitant reduction in mandible protraction. Linked to headaches and pain.
Lateral pterygoid	Subluxation of mandible and dysfunctional movement between disc and mandible, resulting in clicks and possible locking of jaw. Linked to headaches.
Medial pterygoid	Compression of disc and if unilateral, an increased contralateral deviation of jaw, affecting bite mechanics.
Muscles of tongue, Mylohyoid, Digastric, Geniohyoid	Unilateral or imbalanced tightness of these muscles, which act as a floor to the mouth, can affect contralateral movement of mandible and so affect bite mechanism.

Table 1.2: Effects of muscle restrictions on TMJ movement.

Neck

In this book the neck is defined as the cervical spine and those muscles involved in osteokinematic movements as observed by the position of the head with respect to the body and those arthrokinematic movements at joints which enable the gross movements to occur.

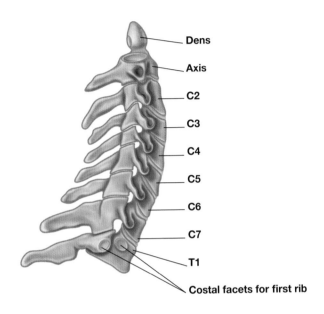

Figure 1.5: Cervical spine and facets.

The articulation between the skull (occipital bone) and the first cervical vertebra is the atlanto-occipital joint; the next articulation, between the first and second vertebrae, is the atlanto-axial joint. Neither of these articulations has a disc. However, the rest of the cervical vertebrae are connected by vertebral discs and facet joints. In addition to these key articulations, C3 to C7 vertebrae also have structures called joints of Luschka and uncinate processes. The way in which these contribute to cervical neck motion is still unclear. It is these various articulations that determine much of the available motion of the neck.

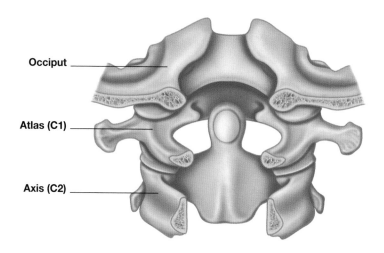

Occiput

Atlas (C1)

Axis (C2)

Figure 1.6: Atlanto-occipital joint.

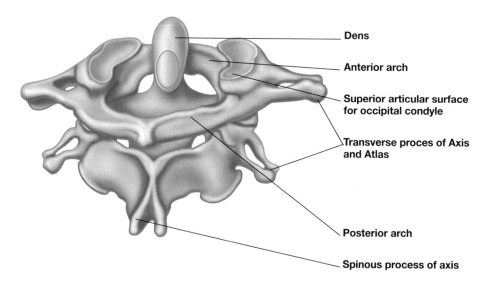

Dens

Anterior arch

Superior articular surface
for occipital condyle

Transverse proces of Axis
and Atlas

Posterior arch

Spinous process of axis

Figure 1.7: Atlanto-axial joint.

Gross (Osteokinematic) Movement of the Neck

The structure of the atlanto-occipital joint provides a high proportion of the flexion and extension movement seen as nodding of the head, whilst the atlanto-axial joint provides almost 50% of rotational movement. The remaining motion of the neck comes from each of the lower cervical joints contributing in part to the full range.

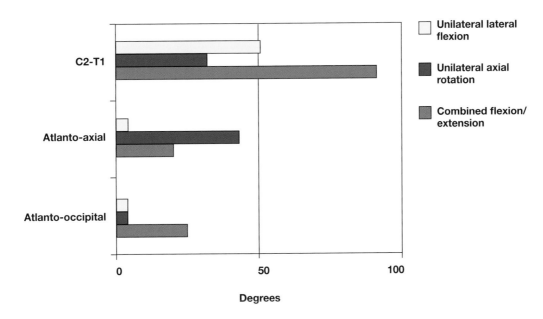

Figure 1.8: Cervical spine segmental range of motion.

Arthrokinematic Movement of the Neck – Coupled Motion

The design of the cervical spine means that motion in one plane does not happen without motion in another; this 'coupled motion' varies as we move down the cervical spine. At the atlanto-occipital joint the occipital condyles translate downwards and backwards as flexion of the head takes place. The atlanto-axial joint does not appear to exhibit defined coupled motion but is responsible for the first 35 to 45 degrees of head rotation before the lower neck moves.

From C2 to C7 (T1) any lateral (side) flexion is accompanied by contralateral rotation (as measured by the spinous process movement). It is now believed that the facet joints and the joints of Luschka are the prime factors in creating coupled motion. Some authors also suggest that extension or flexion motion occurs with lateral and rotational motion as well, although the exact nature of this movement is still unclear. In the lower sections of the cervical spine, flexion is thought to be accompanied by anterior translation and anterior rotation.

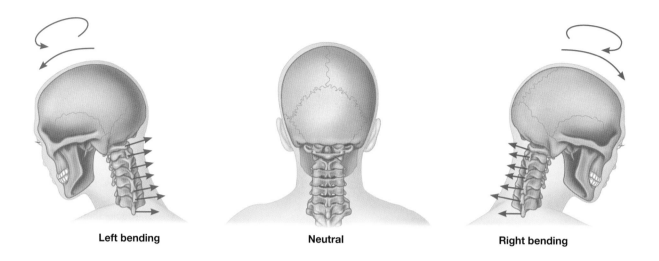

Left bending	Neutral	Right bending

Figure 1.9: Coupled motion C2 to C7.

Muscles of the Neck

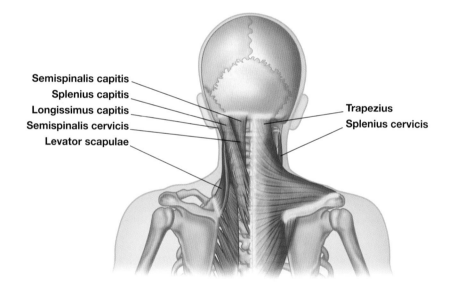

Semispinalis capitis
Splenius capitis
Longissimus capitis
Semispinalis cervicis
Levator scapulae

Trapezius
Splenius cervicis

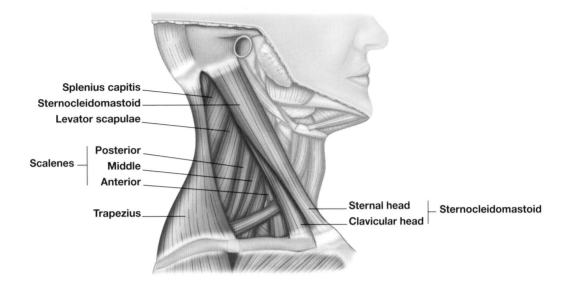

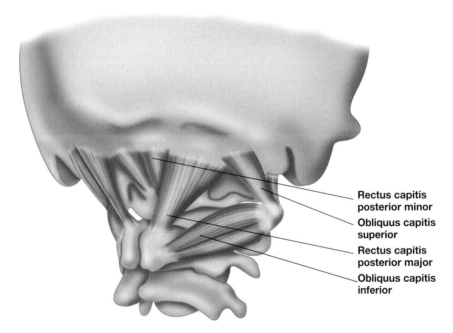

Figure 1.10: Muscles of the neck.

Muscle	Movement of the neck			
	Extension	Flexion	Rotation	Lateral flexion
Suboccipital • Rectus capitis posterior minor • Rectus capitis posterior major • Superior oblique • Inferior oblique	H+CS		H+CS Ipsi	
Semispinalis capitis	H+CS			H+CS
Splenius capitis **(action: head and cervical spine)**	H+CS		H+CS Ipsi	H+CS
Splenius cervicis				
Longissimus capitis	H			H+CS
Levator scapulae **(action: with scapula fixed)**	CS		CS Ipsi	CS
Trapezius **(action with scapula fixed)**			H Contra	H
Sternocleidomastoid		Bi-lateral	H Contra	H Ipsi
Scalenes		CS	H Contra	CS

Key				H	CS	Contra	Ipsi
	Primary role	Secondary role	Possible role	Action on head	Action on cervical spine	Contralateral	Ipsilateral

Table 1.3: Neck muscle movement.

Muscle	Effect of restriction
Suboccipital • Rectus capitis posterior minor • Rectus capitis posterior major • Superior oblique • Inferior oblique	Limited studies exist on the effects of tightness in these muscles, although connections to dura are found in rectus capitis posterior minor, which is associated with headaches. There is also a suggestion that tightness may affect positioning of head, increasing upper cervical extension.
Semispinalis capitis	Reduced flexion of head and cervical spine. Entrapment of greater occipital nerve.
Splenius capitis Splenius cervicis	Reduced flexion of head and cervical spine. Limited studies exist on these muscles.
Longissimus capitis	Increased lateral flexion of head on neck when observed in frontal plane, and posterior rotation of cervical spine.
Levator scapulae	Pain in medial scapula and neck. Increased ipsilateral neck flexion and/or raised scapula.
Trapezius	Reduced head and cervical spine flexion and ipsilateral rotation of head. Head pain is thought to be linked to trigger points in tight upper fibres.
Sternocleidomastoid	Torticollis, both spasmodic and congenital. Head-forward posture. Increased extension of upper cervical spine.
Scalenes	Sensation changes in arms and hands as the brachial plexus is compressed. Reduced rotation and increased lateral flexion of cervical spine.

Table 1.4: Effects of muscle restrictions on neck movement.

Effects of Muscle Restrictions on the Head and Neck in Sport and Everyday Life

Cycling

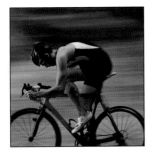

Road cycling requires long periods of head and neck extension. This will often lead to tight sternocleidomastoid (SCM) muscles, and eventually the head and neck extensor muscles will be affected, causing their own problems, including upper back pain and headaches. Not only will this have an impact on cycling performance but it can increase the danger factor, as the ability to rotate the head and neck to look behind will be impaired.

Archery

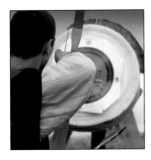

Archery requires the head to be rotated and held at almost full rotation. This is accompanied in many cases by active lateral flexion to line up the sighting eye. This position requires virtually all of the neck muscles to contract and shorten on one side. Raising of the shooting arm will also shorten the upper trapezius and the levator scapulae on the opposite site. Potential issues include headaches and upper extremity pain, paresthesias, numbness, weakness, fatigability, swelling and discoloration due to compression of the brachial plexus at the scalenes.

Driving

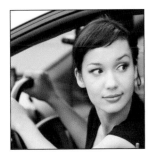

Many people notice neck restrictions for the first time when their ability to rotate their head to look over the shoulder when driving is compromised. This can be caused by tightness in almost any or all of the head and neck muscles but in particular the upper trapezius, scalenes and SCM. However, the coupled motion that occurs throughout the cervical spine can be affected by many of the smaller muscles, and, since almost 50% of rotation occurs at the atlanto-axial joint, restrictions in the muscles of attachment here can also drastically reduce head rotation.

Soft Tissue Release to the Head and Neck

Make a note of the subject's head and neck position. Check his active ROM: flexion/extension, rotation and side flexion.

Be acutely aware of the structures – nerves, arteries and glands – during STR to the muscles of the neck. Be particularly sensitive in the anterior triangle and lock in carefully, addressing muscle borders where possible. When working on the anterior and medial scalenes, the brachial plexus may be compressed if the muscles are congested: avoid too much pressure and work delicately to minimise irritation of the nerve. If the pulse from the carotid artery is felt while grasping the SCM, release immediately and relocate the lock. It is generally advisable for the massage therapist to perform STR actively in the neck region: this will ensure that the subject is moving within a functionally-capable ROM. If the tissue is particularly fibrous or if the ROM is significantly reduced, resisted STR is beneficial.

STR to the sternocleidomastoid (SCM) in supine:

1) With the subject's head in neutral position, gently grasp either side of the SCM; only perform STR on one SCM at a time. Ask him to slowly extend his head. Do the same thing on the other side. If it is difficult to locate the muscle, ask the subject to lift his head off the table and gently grasp the contracting muscle as he places his head back down onto the couch; ask him to extend his head.

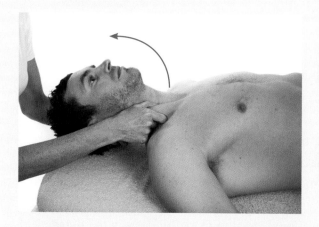 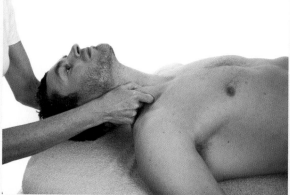

2) Ask the subject to move his head into side flexion and gently grasp the SCM on the shortened side. Ask him to side flex his head the other way for a stretch.

3) With the head in neutral position, gently grasp the SCM; ask him to rotate to the same side for a stretch. Perform locks, starting at the insertion towards the mastoid process, in the belly of the muscle, and two separate locks for the sternal point of origin and the clavicular point of origin.

- It will be easier to do active STR to avoid holding the heavy weight of the head and to avoid moving the neck beyond a comfortable appropriate range.

- Use a CTM lock to pick up the borders of the SCM; try moving each side in the opposite direction, prior to initiating the stretch.

- If the SCM is particularly 'embedded' or difficult to grasp, try addressing the medial and lateral sides one side at a time, rather than grasping the whole muscle.

STR to the anterior, medius and posterior scalenes in supine:

1) Support the subject's head with one hand and gently apply a CTM into the anterior scalenus; apply the lock close to the clavicle and just underneath the lateral border of the SCM, as he inhales. Slowly side flex the neck to the opposite side as he exhales. Apply a lock lateral to this for the medius scalenus.

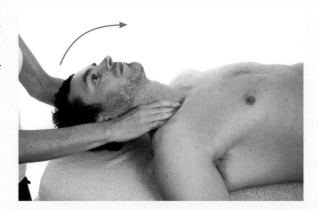

2) Support the head with one hand and side flex the neck, to shorten the muscle, as the subject inhales. Use two fingers to drop into the posterior scalenus, between the medius scalenus and the levator scapulae; side flex away as he exhales.

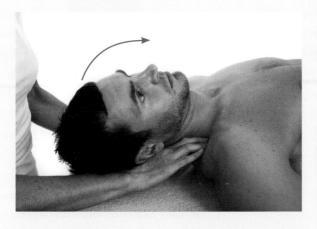
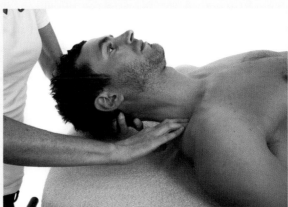

- Compression of the brachial plexus can be caused by restriction to the medius and anterior scalenes – the muscles that this network of nerves runs between. STR is an ideal way of releasing the muscles without causing irritation to the nerves.

STR to the trapezius in supine:

1) Use a phalange or a thumb reinforced with fingers to lock into the trapezius close to C7. Ask the subject to side flex his head to the opposite side. Re-apply a lock in the belly of the muscle and close to the acromion. Ask him to side flex to the opposite side.

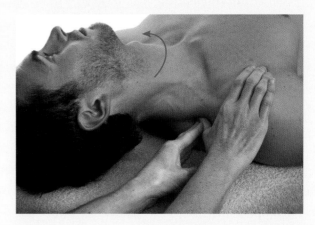

2) Use fingers or a reinforced thumb to lock in close to C7 and ask the subject to slowly side flex his head. This may be easier to do one side at a time while supporting the head on the other side. Apply locks in and away from the ligamentum nuchae; each time ask him to side flex his head.

3) Use a CTM lock on the occiput attachment and ask him to side flex his head.

STR to the trapezius in seated:

1) Hook both hands over the top of the anterior fibres of the upper trapezius and use fingers to curl underneath one side at a time in a CTM lock; ask the subject to alternate between side flexion and rotation of the head. Side flex away from the lock and rotate to the same side for a stretch.

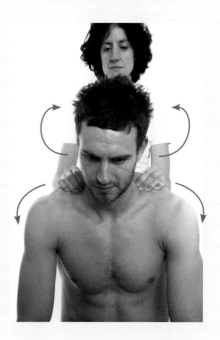

2) Sit on the side of the couch and use fingers to curl under the anterior fibres of the trapezius; ask him to rotate his head to the same side or side flex his head to the opposite side.

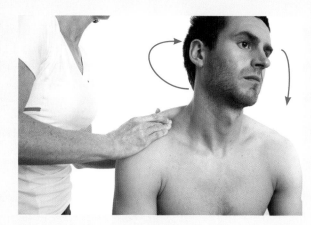

3) Use an elbow or a knuckle to lock in close to C7; ask the subject to flex his neck forwards or to side flex the head to the opposite side. Lock into the belly of the muscle and close to the acromion.

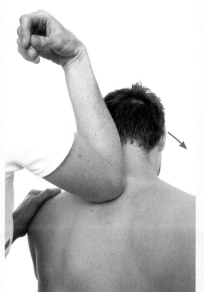

4) Use a CTM lock on the spine of the scapula and ask him to side flex his neck. (See page 63 for release with scapula movement.)

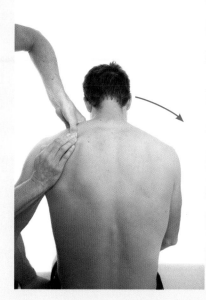

STR to the levator scapulae in seated:

1) Ensure that the upper fibres of the trapezius are warmed up. With a reinforced thumb, lock deep to the trapezius fibres towards the tendon of origin at the superior angle of the scapula. If the anterior fibres of the trapezius are sufficiently free, use fingers to hook underneath them, towards the anterior surface of the superior angle of the scapula. Ask the subject to side flex his neck to the opposite side, or to flex it. For more lengthening ask him to side flex his neck and from that position ask him to flex his neck.

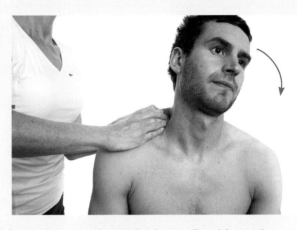

STR to the levator scapulae in supine:

1) Support the side of the subject's head with one hand and use a finger reinforced with another one to curl under the trapezius at C4 level; ask him to side flex his neck gently into the hand. Perform another lock and stretch higher up.

STR to the splenius capitis and splenius cervicis in supine:

1) Lock into the splenius capitis, directly palpable between the SCM and the trapezius, running obliquely to the trapezius, using a finger reinforced with another one. Ask the subject to rotate his head to the opposite side or ask him to tuck his chin in. Use a CTM lock close to the mastoid process.

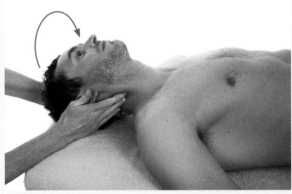

2) Use a thumb reinforced with fingers to lock deep into the splenius muscles close to C7. Ask the subject to rotate his head to the opposite side.

- The splenius cervicis lies deep to the capitis.

STR to the splenius capitis and splenius cervicis in seated:

1) Use the olecranon or a knuckle to lock in deep to the trapezius and close to C7; ask the subject to flex his head forwards or to rotate it to the opposite side. Apply a lock away from the lower half of the ligamentum nuchae and away from the upper three thoracic vertebrae.

2) Use fingers to grasp either side of the trapezius in the cervical region and to curl around its lateral border to target the splenius muscles. Ask the subject to flex his neck. Use a reinforced finger to address one side at a time and ask him to side flex his neck.

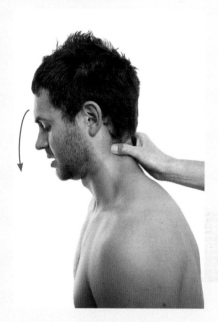

STR to the splenius capitis and splenius cervicis in side lying:

1) Use the index finger reinforced with the middle finger to lock in close to C7; ask the subject to flex his head forwards. He can also try to rotate his head to the other side for resisted STR, by gently pushing his head into the pillow. Apply locks from the lower half of the ligamentum nuchae and away from the upper three thoracic vertebrae.

2) Use a finger to gently lock into the splenius, directly palpable between the trapezius and the SCM; ask the subject to tuck his chin in.

3) Use a CTM lock to address the attachment at the mastoid process; ask him to tuck his chin in.

STR to the erector spinae (spinalis cervicis, longissimus capitis, longissimus cervicis and iliocostalis cervicis) in side lying:

1) Use reinforced fingers to apply locks deep to the trapezius and splenius muscles and close to the spinous processes; ask him to flex his neck forwards. He can also try to side flex his neck by pushing his head down into the pillow.

- Locks can be performed from T7 up to C2.

STR to the transversospinales (semispinalis cervicis and capitis, and multifidus) in supine:

1) Sit or stand at the head of the couch. Use a middle finger reinforced with the index finger to apply a deep pressure into the lamina groove; ask him to tuck his chin in. Apply locks in the cervical region between the transverse and spinous processes.

- Ensure that the more superficial neck muscles of the trapezius, splenius and erector spinae have been loosened up prior to STR in this area.

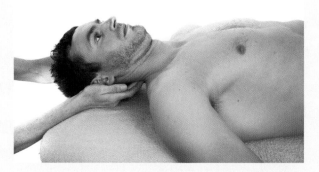

STR to the suboccipitals (rectus capitis posterior major, rectus capitis posterior minor, oblique capitis superior and oblique capitis inferior) in supine:

1) Gently hold the head with both hands and curl fingers underneath the occiput. Slowly lock in deep to the trapezius, splenius capitis and the semispinalis capitis. Ask the subject to slowly tuck his chin in. Slowly lock in away from C1 and lock in away from C2, each time guiding him into a chin tuck.

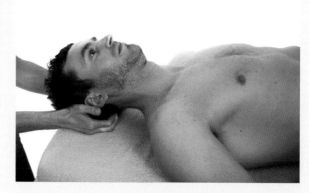

- If the head feels too heavy to do both sides at the same time, support the head with one hand and let the hand rest on the couch; do one side at a time.

STR to the muscles of the TMJ in supine:

It is useful to palpate both sides at the same time during warm-up STR; this allows for a good comparison to be made of both tissue texture and movement of the jaw on each side. To work more specifically and intraorally, treat one side at a time.

1) Use fingers to lock into the temporalis; ask the subject to open his mouth (depress the mandible). Use a CTM lock to address the tendon of origin at the coronoid process; ask him to open his mouth.

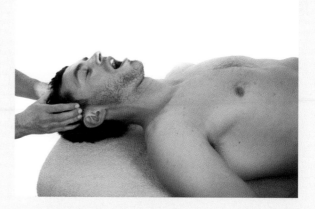

2) Use one finger reinforced with another to lock into the superficial belly of the masseter; ask the subject to open his mouth. The deep belly is palpable from inside the mouth. Use the index finger of each hand to target the muscle from both sides: one locating inside the mouth and the other outside. Ask him to open his mouth.

3) The pterygoids are palpable from both inside and outside of the mouth. Working intraorally provides an effective release. Use the index finger of each hand to target the lateral pterygoid muscle from both sides. Carefully lock in so that the two fingers meet and ask the subject to slowly close his mouth, avoiding any biting of the therapist's finger! Locate the medial pterygoid in the same way and ask him to open his mouth.

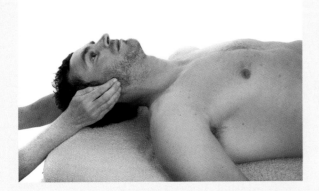 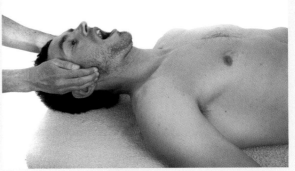

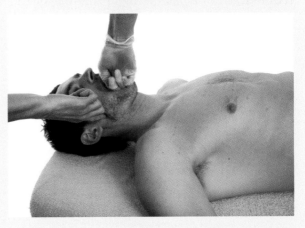

The Shoulder Girdle Complex

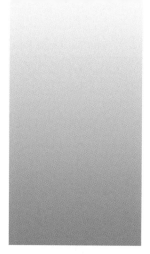

When evaluating the shoulder, the emphasis must always be on the whole shoulder girdle complex and not simply on the 'shoulder', or glenohumeral joint. The shoulder girdle comprises the sternoclavicular, acromioclavicular, glenohumeral and scapulothoracic joints, associated muscles, ligaments and other soft tissue. Its design allows a large ROM, coupled with the requirement of a stable base for muscles to anchor onto. It is a design that enables us to achieve powerful movements necessary in throwing a cricket ball at 100 mph or lifting 200 kg overhead as readily as the intricate control required in throwing a dart or playing the violin.

Limitations in any of the soft tissue components of the shoulder girdle will eventually lead to abnormal movement and the potential for pain and disability at worst and reduced performance at the least. Although the capsule and the ligaments can be a source of restriction, the focus here is on muscular and tendinous tissue restrictions. The shoulder girdle utilises approximately 16 interdependent muscles, and the glenohumeral joint has the greatest ROM of any joint in the body.

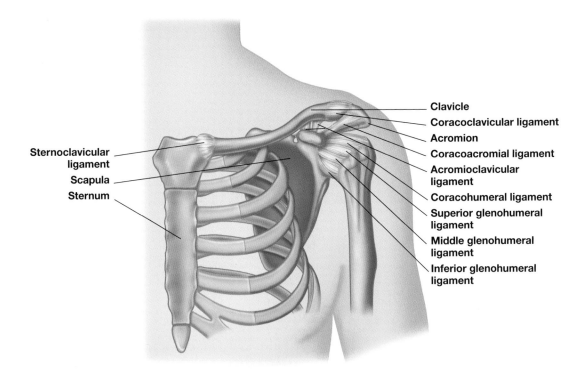

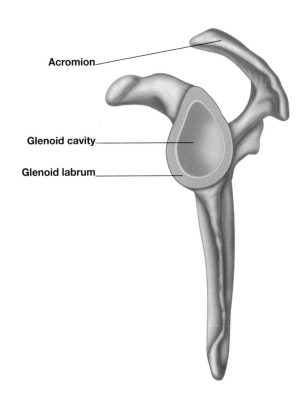

Figure 2.1: Shoulder girdle complex.

Movements of the Shoulder Girdle Complex

There are a number of fundamental gross movements (osteokinematics) associated with the shoulder girdle complex. These movements are normally measured or observed via the location of the arm with respect to the trunk and represent the ROM at the glenohumeral joint. However, underlying these movements are the arthrokinematics at joint surfaces and the gross movements of the scapula and clavicle. These individual movements, which are the result of a complex pattern of muscle activation, combine to create a multitude of integrated patterns of movement that give the shoulder girdle its ability to provide stability with flexibility.

The following section examines the basic gross movements and the arthrokinematics at the associated joints, along with the muscles involved and essential integrated patterns of movement used in clinical settings to identify potential issues.

Gross Observational Movements

Flexion	External humeral rotation
Extension	Internal humeral rotation
Lateral flexion (abduction)	Adduction

Table 2.1: Movements of the glenohumeral joint.

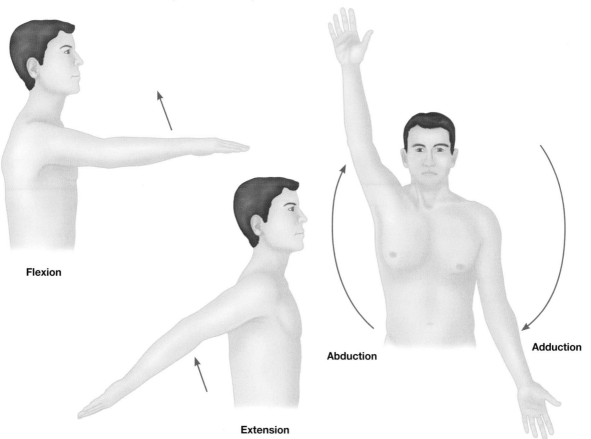

Flexion

Extension

Abduction

Adduction

Protraction (abduction)	Elevation	Upward rotation
Retraction (adduction)	Depression	Downward rotation

Table 2.2: Movements of the scapula.

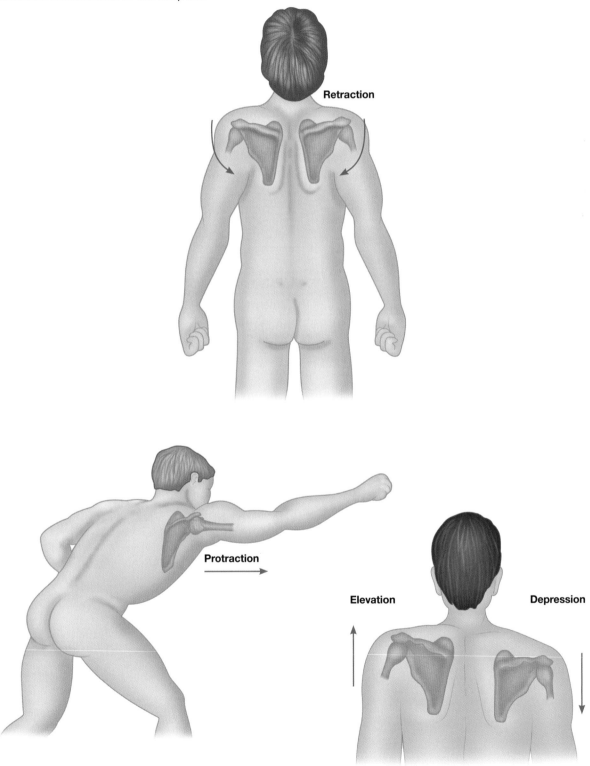

Figure 2.2: Shoulder girdle movement.

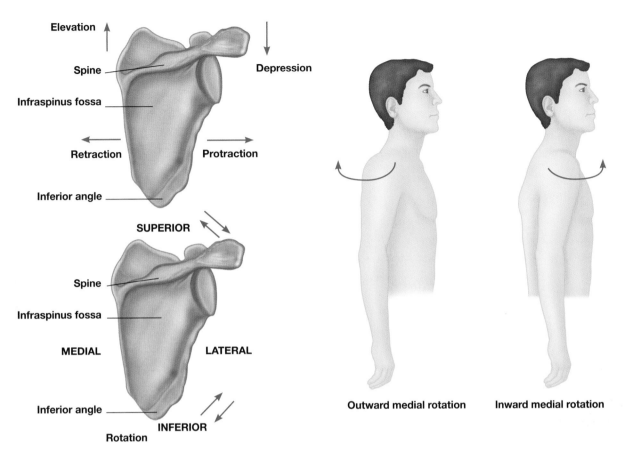

Figure 2.3: Scapular motion.

Elevation	Downward rotation (axial rotation)	Protraction
Depression	Upward rotation	Retraction

Table 2.3: Movement of the clavicle.

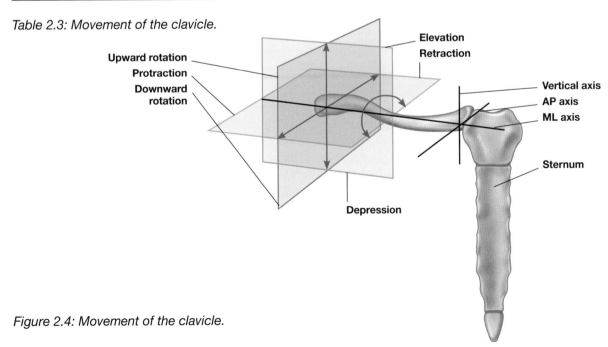

Figure 2.4: Movement of the clavicle.

Apart from depression of the clavicle by the subclavius muscle, movement of the clavicle is determined by its relationship with the movements of the shoulder girdle as a whole. However, restrictions in attached muscles will affect its ability to move as required for full function of the shoulder girdle.

Essential Arthrokinematic Movement

Arthrokinematic movements are those that take place at the joint surfaces and are key to the overall gross movements.

- **Glenohumeral** – between the humeral head and the scapula's glenoid fossa. For the humerus to be abducted in the plane of the scapula (lateral flexion), the humeral head must also translate downwards and laterally (externally) rotate. If either of these does not happen, signs of impingement are seen and felt as the contents of the subacromial space are compressed by the head of the humerus.

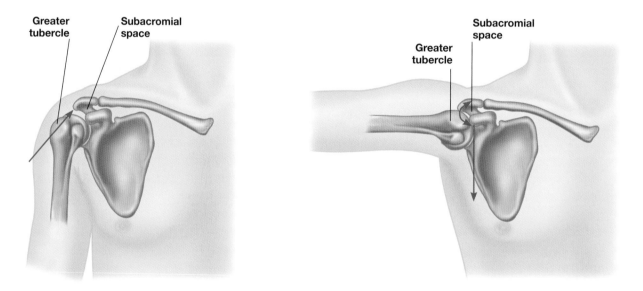

Figure 2.5: Glenohumeral joint arthrokinematics.

- **Sternoclavicular** – between the sternum and the clavicle. Movement of the clavicle is dependent on the arthrokinematics taking place at the sternal notch and the clavicular head. Protraction of the clavicle occurs with posterior roll and anterior movement of the clavicular head; retraction occurs with posterior rotation of the clavicular head and anterior movement of the body.

Integrated Movements

Scapulohumeral Rhythm

Raising the arm laterally – an essential gross movement – depends on the arthrokinematics at the glenohumeral joint, along with movement of the scapula and clavicle. The key pattern observed is known as 'scapulohumeral rhythm'; without this function, the total movement of the shoulder girdle is impossible. The scapula should move approximately in a 1:2 ratio with the humerus in lateral flexion in the scapula plane. The scapula thus provides 60 degrees of upward rotation and the glenohumeral joint 120 degrees to make the full 180 degrees. Although there is a difference of opinion regarding the exact ratio, there is agreement that a pattern exists and can be used by clinicians to identify abnormal patterns of movement.

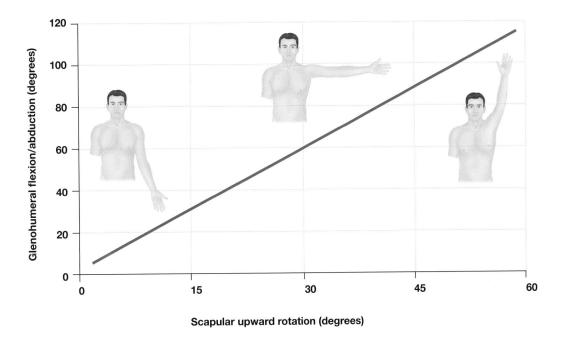

Figure 2.6: Scapulohumeral rhythm.

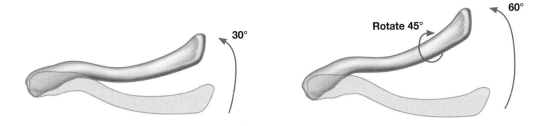

Figure 2.7: Clavicular rotation.

With an upward rotation of the scapula there must also be a concomitant upward elevation of the clavicle: this is approximately 40 degrees for a scapular rotation of 60 degrees. At the same time, the clavicle must also rotate posteriorly to utilise its crank shape to increase movement.

Essential Muscle Synergies for Movement

As part of the integrated movement of the shoulder girdle, groups of muscles work in synergy to provide 'force couples'. Restrictions in any of these muscles will affect these balancing force couples. This will prompt abnormal compensatory movements to occur, having long-term effects on associated structures, which then lead to pathology and reduced performance.

The upward rotation of the scapula requires the upper trapezius to work in tandem with the lower trapezius, and for total humeral-trunk elevation the serratus anterior must balance the whole of the trapezius muscle.

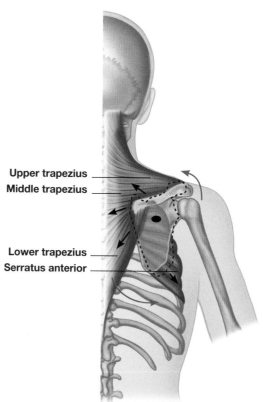

Figure 2.8: Trapezius-serratus relationship.

Downward rotation of the scapula is created by the pull of the levator scapulae along with the rhomboids, which would create adduction of the scapula without the balancing effect of the pectoralis minor muscle.

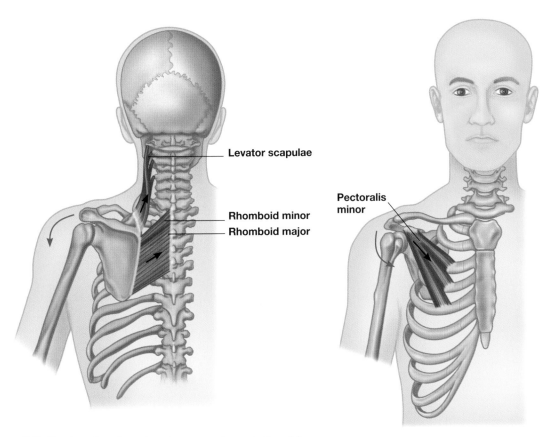

Figure 2.9: Pectoralis minor-levator scapulae relationship.

The rotator cuff muscles work with the deltoid in the frontal plane and with each other in the transverse plane. They act to stabilise the joint as movement is initiated and the arm abducted.

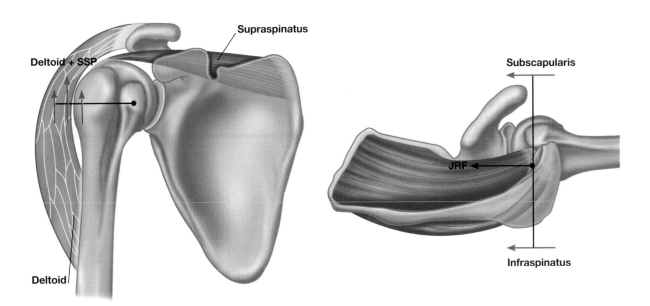

Figure 2.10: Deltoid-supraspinatus (SSP) relationship.

Figure 2.11: Rotator cuff relationship, the joint reaction force (JRF) of both muscles working together.

Shoulder Girdle Muscles

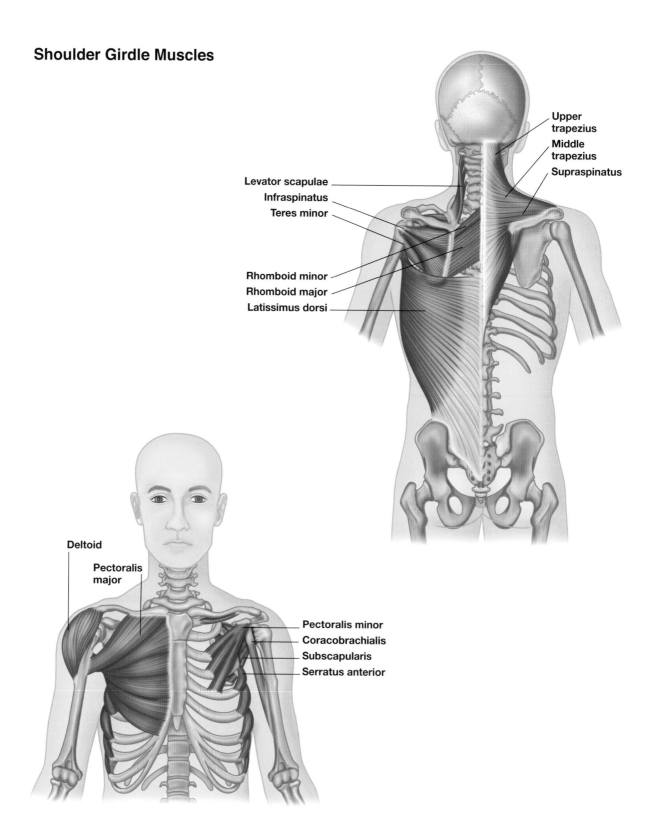

Figure 2.12: Shoulder girdle muscles.

Muscle	Movement of the humerus					
	Lateral flexion (abduction)	Anterior flexion	Extension	Internal (medial) rotation	External (lateral) rotation	Adduction
Pectoralis major (clavicular)		Primary		Primary		Primary
Pectoralis major (sterno)				Primary		Primary
Deltoid (anterior)	Primary	Primary		Primary		
Deltoid (medial)	Primary					
Deltoid (posterior)	Primary		Primary		Primary	
Infraspinatus	Primary				Primary	
Teres major			Primary	Primary		Primary
Teres minor	Possible				Primary	
Supraspinatus	Secondary					
Subscapularis				Primary		
Coracobrachialis		Primary				
Latissimus dorsi			Primary	Primary		Secondary
Triceps			Primary			
Biceps		Primary				

Muscle	Movement of the scapula					
	Protraction (abduction	Retraction (adduction)	Depression	Elevation	Upward rotation	Downward rotation
Pectoralis minor	Secondary	Secondary	Secondary	Secondary		
Trapezius (upper)		Primary		Primary	Primary	
Trapezius (middle)		Primary				
Trapezius (lower)		Primary			Primary	Secondary
Levator scapulae				Primary		Primary
Rhomboids		Primary		Primary		Primary
Serratus anterior	Primary				Secondary	
Latissimus dorsi			Primary			

Key	Primary role	Secondary or weak role	Possible role

Table 2.4: Muscle movement at the shoulder girdle.

Effects of Muscle Restrictions on Shoulder Girdle Movement

When muscles are not capable of fulfilling their normal roles, it is often through weakness, tightness, injury or a pathological change brought about by disease. In this book we are concerned with restrictions in muscles and other soft tissues that prevent full movement taking place around a joint complex.

Muscle	Effect of restriction
Pectoralis major	Can limit all ROM in shoulder girdle. Key limitation likely to be found with horizontal abduction and lateral rotation around long axis of humerus. Clavicular head affects lateral rotation, whilst the sternal section is likely to affect shoulder abduction, flexion and lateral rotation. Scapula retraction can be restricted especially with weak scapula retraction muscles.
Pectoralis minor	Impact on the combined motions that result from its force-couple relationship with the levator scapula and rhomboids. Can also lead to thoracic outlet syndrome by compression of the brachial plexus, which runs beneath it. Postural changes associated with 'rounded shoulders'.
Trapezius (upper, middle, lower)	Upper: elevated shoulders and reduced ROM head and neck. Middle: scapula abduction (although rare). Lower: thoracic spine curve at insertion and impact on force couple.
Serratus anterior	Reduced upward rotation of scapula, inability to raise arms fully above head in frontal plane, abnormal scapulohumeral motion and increased stress on glenohumeral joint.
Levator scapulae	Reduced cervical rotation, elevation of medial section upper scapula (appearance of elevated shoulder), and head tilt with lateral flexion of humerus. In conjunction with rhomboids contributes to 'round-shouldered' posture.
Rhomboids	Impact on scapulohumeral rhythm and, along with levator scapulae, development of 'round-shouldered' posture is influenced.
Subclavius	Reduced sternoclavicular joint elevation, impacting on scapulohumeral rhythm.
Deltoid (anterior, medial, posterior)	Anterior section: reduced extension. Medial section: reduced glide during glenohumeral movement with lateral abduction, and increased stress on glenohumeral joint. Posterior section: reduced medial rotation and anterior flexion.
Infraspinatus	Reduced medial rotation and horizontal adduction, and increased stress on glenohumeral joint.

Teres major	Reduced lateral rotation, flexion and abduction, and contribution to 'round-shouldered' posture by increased lateral rotation (upward) of scapula with humerus fixed.
Teres minor	Reduced medial rotation of shoulder. Similar effects to those of infraspinatus, but much reduced.
Supraspinatus	Potential impact on downward translation or position of humeral head with humeral abduction.
Subscapularis	Significant impact on scapulohumeral rhythm, abnormal positioning of humeral head, and decreased lateral rotation and horizontal adduction.
Coracobrachialis	Decreased abduction and extension of shoulder, and tilting of scapula (depression of coracoid process) when arm at side.
Latissimus dorsi	Impeded flexion and lateral rotation of shoulder and flexion of thoracic spine, with implications for position of scapula on ribs.

Table 2.5: Effects of muscle restrictions on the shoulder girdle.

Effects of Shoulder Girdle Restrictions in Sport and Everyday Life

Golf

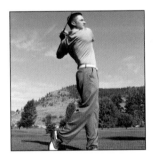

The modern golf swing often tends towards a greater degree of shoulder girdle rotation than in the past. The progress of muscular movement in a golf swing can be summarised as scapulothoracic – glenohumeral – thoracic spine, and then reversed on the downswing and follow-through. Any restriction in the shoulder girdle will reduce performance in two ways. The first is a requirement for greater muscular energy to overcome restriction, which becomes tiring when playing 18 holes. The second is an inability to actually align the upper and lower body for an efficient swing. Even holding the head still to focus on the ball will be impossible without adequate shoulder girdle movement.

It is likely that restrictions in the shoulder girdle will translate down to the low back as the golfer attempts to compensate for reduced shoulder girdle flexibility by way of low back rotation; this may in part explain the prevalence of low back problems.

Phase of swing	Upper body muscles most active
Backswing	Left subscapularis, right upper trapezius
Early downswing	Left rhomboids, right pectoralis major, latissimus dorsi
Acceleration	Pectoralis major bilaterally
Impact	Increased forearm flexor activity, termed the 'flexor burst'
Early follow-through	Pectoralis major bilaterally
Late follow-through	Left infraspinatus, right subscapularis

Source: Adapted from A. McHardy & H. Pollard, 2005, 'Muscle activity during the golf swing', Br. J. Sports Med., 39, pp. 799-804.

Table 2.6: The golf swing.

Swimming

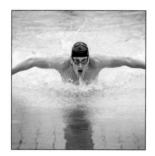

Shoulder impingement problems are common in swimmers. A potential cause is tight pectoral muscles, resulting in the development of a 'round-shouldered' posture. This can lead to an abnormal positioning of the humeral head and an increased chance of acromioclavicular impingement during the overarm stroke.

The basic movement in front crawl involves protraction, and upward rotation of the scapula as a result of strong serratus anterior action. The pectoralis major activates, adducting and extending the humerus, while internal rotation should be balanced by the external rotation of the teres minor. Restriction in any of these muscles will have an impact on the coordinated action required to achieve an efficient stroke.

Brushing Hair

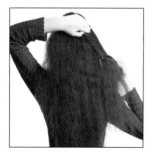

For most people, brushing the hair is a simple task; however, it can be painful (or impossible) to do if there are restrictions in any number of the shoulder girdle muscles. Restriction in the subscapularis will reduce its ability to stabilise the glenohumeral joint and affect the movements which are necessary for holding and moving the arm when brushing the hair. The scapulohumeral rhythm is disrupted, and essential lateral rotation and horizontal adduction of the humerus, necessary for achieving a 'hair brushing' position, is either reduced or impossible. Pain referral patterns into the upper arm are also common.

Soft Tissue Release to the Shoulder Girdle

Make a note of the subject's natural position when standing and when seated. Check through the subject's active ROM, both the shoulder girdle and the shoulder joint. Passive STR is a good way to warm-up the tissues; however, with any area where there is a painful restriction, such as in shoulder rotation, it is advisable to start with active STR. In this case the subject can move comfortably as the therapist slowly guides him through a range of appropriate movement patterns.

It is recommended to perform STR to the shoulder girdle muscles prior to the shoulder joint. Release of restrictions in the shoulder girdle will improve scapular and clavicular movements, as well as improving the range and control of glenohumeral joint movement.

STR to the serratus anterior in side lying:

1) Hold the subject's elbow and grasp between the serratus anterior and the latissimus dorsi by trying to lift the latissimus dorsi slightly; abduct the arm passively. For active STR ask the subject to raise his elbow while keeping his hands together.

   - Ensuring that the serratus anterior is not sticking to the latissimus dorsi will improve scapula movement.

   - Only a small movement may be required.

2) Hold the elbow and apply a CTM lock, using the whole hand, across the surface of the muscle; move the elbow back to retract the scapula. Reinforce the hand and apply a CTM lock; ask the subject to retract his scapula by drawing his elbow back. Use a CTM lock to address the attachments on the anterior surface of the scapula.

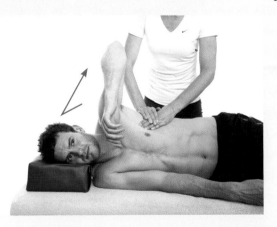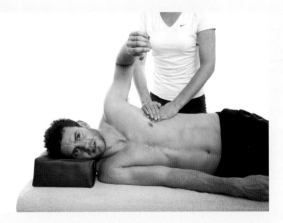

   - Avoid pressing into the ribs; keep the hand relaxed as it melds around the shape of the rib cage.

STR to the serratus anterior in supine:

1) Use a soft fist to apply a CTM lock across the surface of the ribs and into the serratus anterior; ask the subject to retract his scapula and abduct his shoulder.

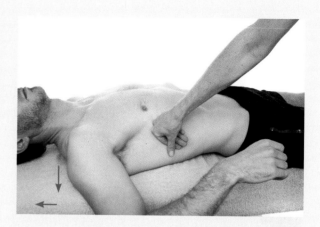

STR to the pectoralis major in supine:

1) With the shoulder at 90 degrees, cup the subject's elbow with one hand. Lock in with the heel of the other hand or knuckles; horizontally abduct the shoulder. Shorten the muscle by horizontally adducting the shoulder prior to the lock, or position the subject at the end of the couch for greater range. Address the sternal attachments with a CTM lock using one or two phalanges.

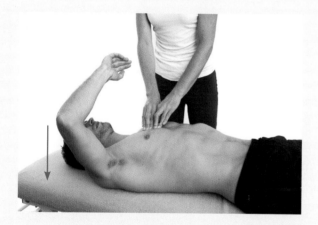 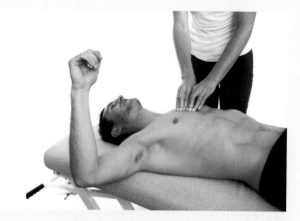

- Even on larger-muscled people this can be a sensitive area to work, so check your speed!

- STR through clothing or towels is useful when treating females.

2) With the shoulder at 90 degrees, gently take hold of the subject's hand and lock into the clavicular fibres with a soft fist; laterally rotate the shoulder.

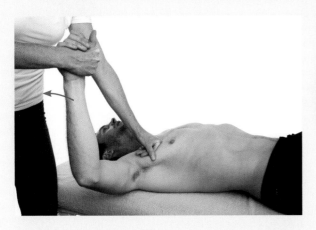 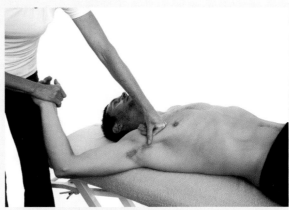

3) Gently grasp the pectoralis major towards the insertion; ask the subject to flex or horizontally adduct the shoulder. Apply a CTM lock at the bicipital groove insertion; direct the subject into a minimal stretch.

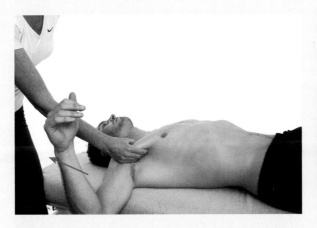 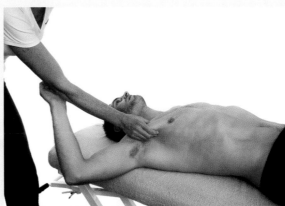

STR to pectoralis minor in supine:

1) Prior to treatment, ensure that the pectoralis major has been 'released'. Use broad surface knuckles, or fingers, to drop in off the coracoid process. Ask the subject to actively retract the scapula into the couch.

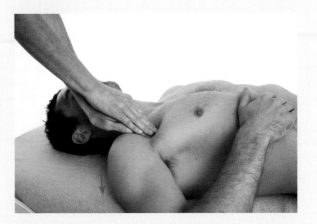

2) Slowly direct fingers underneath the pectoralis major towards the third rib attachment and guide the subject to retract the scapula. Repeat, directing fingers towards the fifth rib.

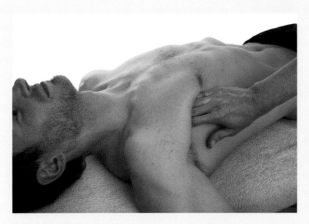 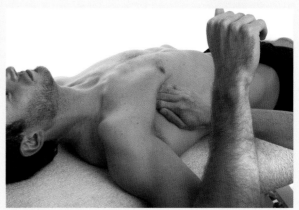

- Do not force through resistant tissue. Move slowly to reach the pectoralis minor fibres. Stop before reaching the muscle if there is too much tissue congestion and perform STR at that level.

STR to subclavius in supine:

1) Use the first phalange to direct a CTM lock down from the clavicle. Ask the subject to elevate his scapula.

STR to the lower fibres of the trapezius in prone:

1) Hook fingers under the border of the lower trapezius and ask the subject to elevate his shoulder.

- Although this part of the trapezius rarely becomes tight, there are often restrictions at the border. Ensuring that there are no adhesions here will facilitate strengthening programmes targeted at the lower fibres.

STR to upper fibres of trapezius in seated:

1) Gently grasp the upper fibres of the trapezius; ask the subject to slowly depress his scapula.

2) Ask the subject to shorten the muscle first by shrugging his shoulder. As he does so, support the scapula or flexed elbow to relax the tissue prior to locking in. Use fingers to lock in; ask him to relax his scapula or to gently push down into the supporting hold.

3) Try a lock close to the acromion, engage the anterior fibres of the upper trapezius, address the spine of the scapula with a CTM lock and apply a lock away from C6/C7.

• See pages 38–39 for STR to upper trapezius with head movement.

STR to upper fibres of trapezius and levator scapulae in prone:

1) Stand at the head of the couch and cup the subject's shoulder with one hand. Lock into the muscle with the heel of the other hand and push the shoulder down to depress the scapula.

2) Still at the head of the couch, liberate both hands and use a reinforced thumb to drop into the muscle. Ask the subject to slide his hand down the side of his leg to depress the scapula.

3) From the side of the couch, cup the subject's anterior shoulder with one hand and use the fingers of the other hand to hook into the muscle; pull the shoulder down into depression.

• Do not force the shoulder into medial rotation if there is any restriction in this movement.

4) Stand at the head of the couch. With one thumb reinforced with the other, lock in deep to the upper trapezius towards the insertion of the levator scapulae at the superior medial angle of the scapula; ask the subject to slide his hand down the side of his leg to depress the scapula.

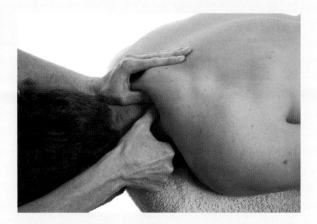

STR to levator scapulae in seated:

1) Ensure that the upper fibres of the trapezius are warmed up. Grasp the lower angle of the scapula with one hand and elevate the scapula. Use fingers or a reinforced phalange to apply a deep pressure towards the levator scapulae at the attachment of the anterior superior angle of the scapula. Gently depress the scapula.

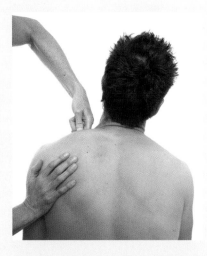

2) The same can be done by directing the lock underneath the anterior fibres of the trapezius. This can be painful so it is essential to work slowly. Do not force through a restriction.

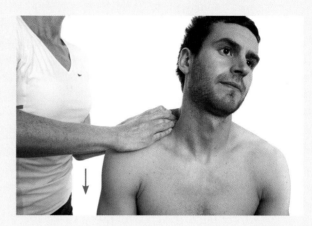

- Make sure that the upper fibres of the trapezius are 'released' prior to working on the levator scapulae.

- See page 40 for further STR on the levator scapulae with neck movement.

STR to the upper fibres of the trapezius and the levator scapulae in side lying:

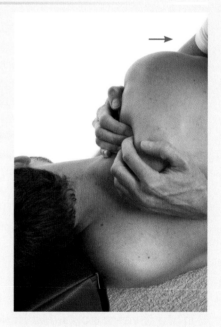

1) Use fingers to lock into the fibres of the upper trapezius and depress the scapula by gently pulling it down.

STR to middle fibres of the trapezius and rhomboids in seated:

1) Support the subject's clavicle and use a gentle fist, the heel of the hand or an elbow to lock into the muscle with a broad surface lock. Instruct the subject to move his arm forwards, or across his body, to protract and rotate the scapula as necessary.

2) Use a knuckle, a reinforced thumb, fingers or an elbow to apply a deeper lock. Lock in and away from the medial border of the scapula. Lock in and away from the spinous processes. Ask him to protract his scapula.

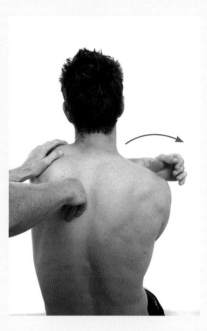

- Vary the direction or the lock. Consider the direction of the fibres of the trapezius, running in a 'V' from the spinous processes (C7–T6) to the scapula, and of the deeper rhomboids (C7–T5), running obliquely to them.

- Vary the arm movement to facilitate a particular movement of the scapula, from miniscule protraction of the scapula with the arm fixed, to broad arm movements across the front or the body.

STR to middle fibres of trapezius and rhomboids in prone:

1) In prone position, subtle CTM locks can be used to lock away from the vertical border of the scapula as it is actively protracted into the couch. Careful 'reading' of the tissue in deciding the direction, depth and speed while attaining the lock will provide a fast release, even with minimal movement of the scapula.

- For a greater ROM, try positioning the subject on the edge of the couch so that he can move his arm underneath it, to protract his scapula.

STR to the middle fibres of trapezius and rhomboids in side lying:

1) Use a thumb reinforced with the other to apply a lock into the muscle. Ask the subject to move his arm into horizontal adduction to protract the scapula.

- This is a good position for progressing to release of the deeper erector spinae muscles.

STR to the deltoids in seated:

1) Position the subject at the end of the couch and stand facing his middle deltoid. Ask him to abduct the shoulder to 90 degrees. Grasp his whole upper arm and use a thumb reinforced with the other one to lock into the medial fibres, drawing down and away from the clavicle. Ask him to adduct his shoulder.

2) Stand behind the couch to engage the posterior fibres away from the clavicle as the subject flexes his shoulder; stand in front to engage the anterior fibres as the subject extends his shoulder. Keep the elbow flexed for ease of movement.

STR to the deltoids in side lying:

1) Stand at the head of the couch. Ask the subject to abduct his shoulder while his elbow remains flexed. Grasp the shoulder with both hands and lock in, with a reinforced thumb, away from the clavicle into the medial fibres of the deltoid. Maintain the lock as the subject adducts his shoulder.

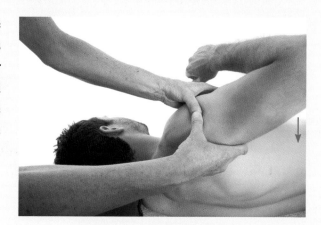

2) Stand at the side of the couch. Gently hook fingers into the fibres of the anterior deltoid and direct it towards the deltoid tuberosity. Ask the subject to extend his shoulder while the elbow remains flexed. Lock into the anterior fibres and ask the subject to laterally rotate his shoulder.

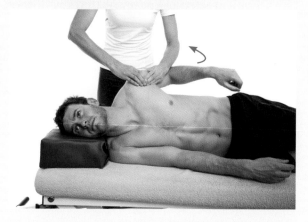

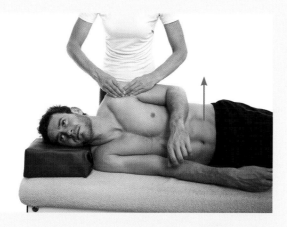
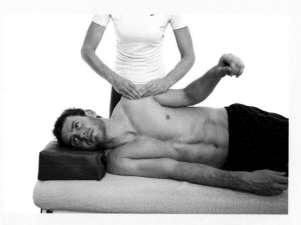

3) Use a reinforced thumb to engage the posterior fibres of the deltoid; ask the subject to flex his shoulder while the elbow remains flexed.

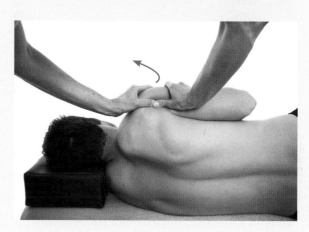

STR to the anterior deltoid in supine:

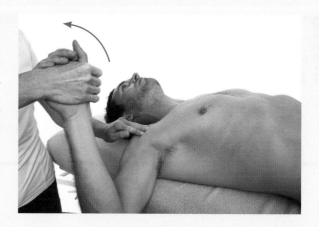

1) Stand at the head of the couch and grasp the subject's hand, with the elbow and shoulder both at 90 degrees. Use fingers to apply a traversing lock into the anterior deltoid and laterally rotate the shoulder. This can be done actively, but passive STR here does provide a very relaxing release.

• Do not go too deep with the lock.

STR to the supraspinatus in prone:

1) Ensure that the upper fibres of the trapezius have been released. Stand at the head of the couch with the subject's shoulder at 90 degrees. Use one thumb reinforced with the other to slowly apply a deep lock, through the trapezius muscle and into the supraspinatus. Ask the subject to adduct his shoulder.

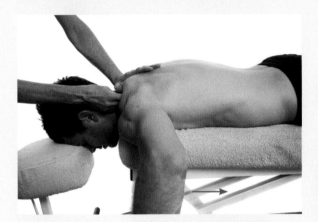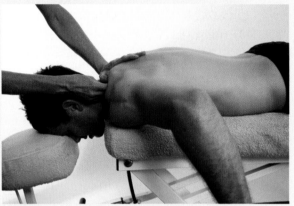

- Try a lock close to the acromion and one closer to the superior angle of the scapula.

STR to the supraspinatus in seated:

1) Ensure that the upper fibres of the trapezius have been released. Ask the subject to abduct his shoulder to 90 degrees. Cup fingers on top of the trapezius; reinforce them with the fingers of the other hand and slowly apply a deep lock into the supraspinatus. Ask the subject to adduct his shoulder.

- Avoid crushing into the tissue: try 'tweezing' in with the fingertips. If the trapezius is too dense to acquire a lock in a shortened position, do not abduct the shoulder first. Perform STR with a minimal stretch by asking the subject to adduct his shoulder by pushing his arm into his side.

2) Use a CTM lock to drop inferiorly off the acromion, deep to the deltoid fibres, onto the surface of the tendon insertion; ask him to adduct his shoulder into his side.

- Putting the shoulder in medial rotation exposes the tendon, making it easier to locate.

STR to the infraspinatus and teres minor in prone:

1) Stand at the head of the couch with the subject's shoulder at 90 degrees. Apply a CTM lock with a reinforced thumb or fingers across the fibres of the infraspinatus. Ask the subject to medially rotate his shoulder. Perform three or four locks here, ensuring that one is performed close to the insertion point at the greater tubercle (deep to the posterior deltoid).

- This is a very sensitive area and locking into the muscle will often produce a trigger point. Do not rush, and give the subject a break between each lock.

STR to the subscapularis in supine:

1) Stand at the side of the couch with the subject's arm horizontally abducted to 90 degrees and the elbow flexed. Use fingers reinforced with the other hand to slowly attain a CTM lock into the subscapularis on the anterior surface of the scapula. Ask the subject to laterally rotate his shoulder.

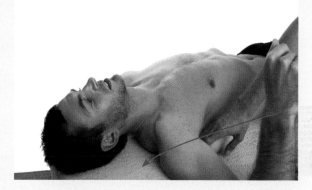

2) With his arm by his side, apply a CTM lock to the tendon of insertion. Lock away from the lesser tubercle (in between the two biceps tendons and deep to the anterior deltoids); ask him to laterally rotate his shoulder.

STR to the latissimus dorsi and teres major in side lying:

1) Gently grasp the borders of the latissimus dorsi where it converges towards the humerus. Ask the subject to abduct his shoulder.

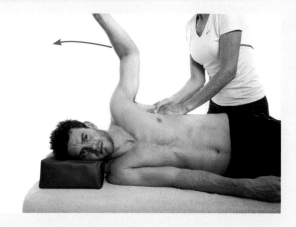
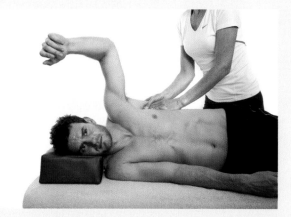

- Ensure that a lock is performed close to the origin on the inferior angle of the scapula as this will help facilitate scapula movement.

- On people with a flexible latissimus dorsi, it is hard to feel a local lengthening. Try to feel the border of the latissimus dorsi and add in some lateral rotation for more stretch (ask the subject to try to place his hand on his head).

2) Perform locks all the way down to the lumbar spine. Use fingers to curl under the lateral border of the muscle, and use CTM locks to engage the thoracolumbar fascia.

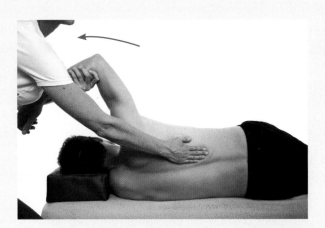

- Try working close to the posterior iliac crest.

- During shoulder abduction, try to feel the tissues moving when locked in at the origins on the lower three ribs.

3) Engage the muscle and guide the subject into active shoulder abduction. A more precise stretch will be obtained by keeping the elbow flexed and the hands together on the couch while active abduction is performed.

- Try using a CTM lock at the origin on the scapula.

- This is a great position for addressing the insertion. Consider the teres major along with the latissimus dorsi attachments and add in an active lateral rotation for a further stretch.

STR to the latissimus dorsi and teres major in prone:

1) Use a broad surface lock, such as the whole hand, slightly cupped, or a gentle fist to engage the latissimus dorsi. Ask the subject to abduct his shoulder. Address the scapula attachment and consider the lateral borders of the muscle as well as the muscle belly.

2) Use a knuckle close to the origin at the spinous processes to perform a CTM lock. Ask the subject to abduct his shoulder. Work down from T6 to the iliac crest.

STR to the coracobrachialis and the long and short heads of the biceps brachii in supine:

1) Cup the subject's flexed elbow with one hand or hold the wrist. Lift it up to flex his shoulder and lock fingers into the tendons of the anterior shoulder. Apply a lock across the coracobrachialis, away from the coracoid process, and drop the elbow passively to extend his shoulder. Apply a lock in the same way for the biceps brachii; use a CTM lock to distinguish between the two tendons.

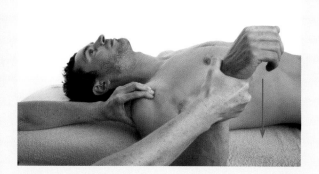

- Try abducting the shoulder to locate the coracobrachialis more easily.

- Try laterally rotating the shoulder to locate the long head of the biceps.

- Position the subject with his shoulder off the side of the couch. Gently tweeze between the tendons as the subject actively extends his shoulder.

STR to the long head of the triceps brachii in side lying:

Grasp the subject's flexed elbow with one hand. Lock in away from the origin of the long head of the triceps; move the shoulder into flexion.

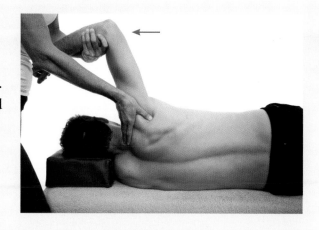

The Elbow

3

As part of the upper limb the elbow joint has muscles common to both the shoulder and the wrist and must be examined in a clinical setting as part of that chain. Restriction of a common muscle may have a completely different effect on elbow movement when compared to either the shoulder or the wrist.

The elbow joint is formed from the humerus connecting with the ulna and radius of the forearm. It has a capsule and lateral and medial collateral ligaments. The structure of the distal humerus and proximal radius and ulna makes the elbow joint more than a simple hinge joint and it is sometimes described as a trochoginglymus joint.

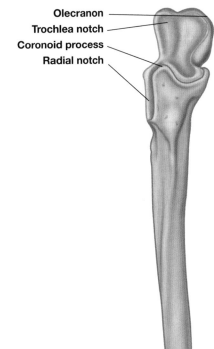

Olecranon
Trochlea notch
Coronoid process
Radial notch

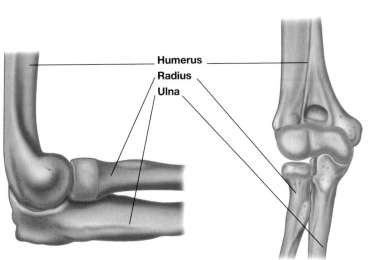

Humerus
Radius
Ulna

Figure 3.1: Structure of the elbow.

Movement of the Elbow Joint

As a trochoginglymus joint the elbow complex is capable of flexion and extension, as well as some medial and lateral rotation at the humeral surfaces. Pronation and supination are the other key movements at the elbow, although these occur at the radioulnar joint.

Maximum flexion is generally in the range of 140 to 150 degrees. Extension can sometimes become hyperextension, but in the general population this is limited, although people with hypermobility syndrome often have markedly increased hyperextension of the elbow. Flexion and extension seem to occur around a fixed axis, although some studies suggest that the carrying angle decreases as flexion occurs.

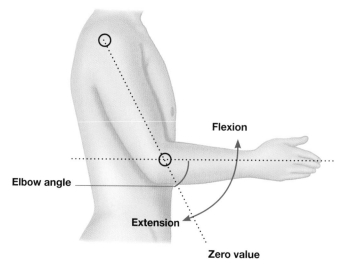

Figure 3.2: Elbow range of motion.

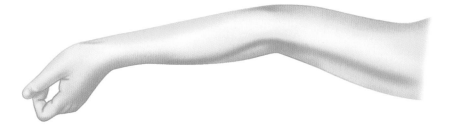

Figure 3.3: Elbow hyperextension.

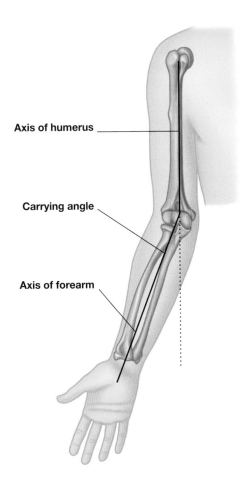

Axis of humerus

Carrying angle

Axis of forearm

Figure 3.4: Carrying angle.

Pronation and supination in their basic forms involve relative rotation of the ulna and radius. The ulna appears fixed, with the distal radius moving around it. The axis of motion is considered fixed and passes through the line of the radial fovea. Evidence is weak for additional motion in supination and pronation, although there is a suggestion of a more complicated compound motion at the ulna.

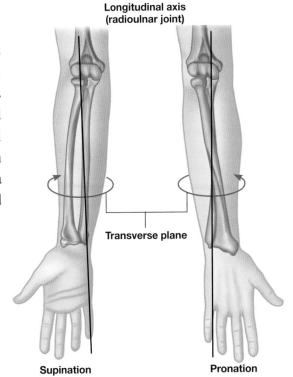

**Longitudinal axis
(radioulnar joint)**

Transverse plane

Supination

Pronation

Figure 3.5: Pronation and supination.

The Elbow Muscles

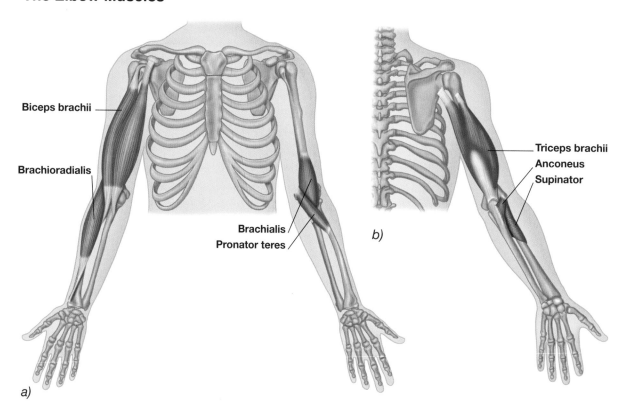

Figure 3.6: Elbow joint muscles; a) anterior view, b) posterior view.

Muscle	Movement of the elbow			
	Flexion	Extension	Supination	Pronation
Biceps brachii	███		███	
Supinator			███	
Brachialis	███			
Triceps brachii		███		
Brachioradialis	███		░░░	░░░
Anconeus		Weak		
Pronator teres	▓▓▓			▓▓▓

Key	Primary role	Secondary or weak role	Possible role

Table 3.1: Muscle movement at the elbow joint.

Muscle	Effect of restriction
Biceps brachii	Reduced elbow extension and pronation. Because of the two-joint nature of this muscle, tightness will affect the interaction of shoulder and elbow movement. With the shoulder in extension, elbow extension will be reduced; conversely, with the shoulder flexed, the elbow ROM increases.
Brachialis	As a single-joint muscle, elbow extension will be reduced (regardless of shoulder position).
Supinator	Tightness of the supinator is more likely in conjunction with tightness of the biceps brachii rather than by itself, but it would probably reduce elbow extension and pronation.
Triceps brachii	Limited elbow flexion and some reduction in anterior shoulder elevation. Can be implicated in tennis elbow.
Brachioradialis	Reduced elbow extension.
Anconeus	No known effect.
Pronator teres	Loss of elbow flexion and forearm supination. Due to origin and insertion at the elbow joint and the superior distal radioulnar joint, the effect of tightness will depend on the relative positions of these articulations, with reduced supination when the elbow is extended.

Table 3.2: Effects of muscle restrictions on elbow movement.

Effects of Elbow Restrictions in Sport and Everyday Life

Tennis

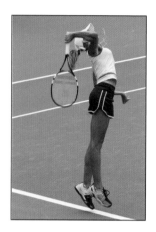

Restriction of the elbow extensors (triceps) can potentially affect tennis performance in a number of ways. It is estimated that the elbow will flex from 120 degrees to 20 degrees in 0.2 seconds at the start of a serve. Any undue tension in the triceps could reduce the ability to take the arm back into the serving position and therefore have an impact on both speed and power of the serve. The action of bringing the racket arm into a backhand position may also be impaired through tightness both at the elbow and at the shoulder, and there may be increased potential for injuries in other areas, for example in the low back, as the trunk is engaged to gain necessary rotation. The follow-through of a serve is often associated with fast and powerful pronation at the elbow and internal rotation at the shoulder. Restriction in the triceps brachii will also impact on this movement, increasing the chance of overuse injury.

Crown Green and Lawn Bowls

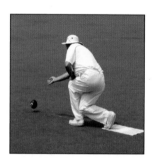

A successful delivery in bowling is dependent on correct arm movement. A biceps restriction would prevent a smooth backswing because of the two-joint nature of the muscle across the shoulder and the elbow. It would also affect the forward delivery by limiting a smooth and full extension at the elbow.

Washing and Dressing

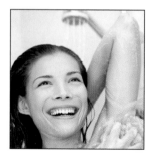

Basic everyday activities can be severely limited by restrictions in both elbow flexors and elbow extensors. Washing the hair and under the arms can be impossible with restricted triceps, as shoulder and elbow flexion would be limited. At worst, even eating becomes difficult. Contracture of the biceps brachii can make putting on a shirt or a coat more difficult.

Soft Tissue Release to the Elbow

Make a note of the presentation of the subject's elbow when standing and when seated. Check ROM through flexion, extension, supination and pronation.

STR to the biceps brachii and brachialis in supine:

1) With the subject's elbow flexed, grasp either side of the belly of the biceps brachii; extend and pronate the elbow, or ask him to extend and pronate the elbow. Use fingers to apply a CTM lock away from the coracoid process into the tendon of the short head and ask the subject to extend and pronate the elbow. Use fingers to lock into the long head in the intertubercular groove; ask him to extend and pronate the elbow.

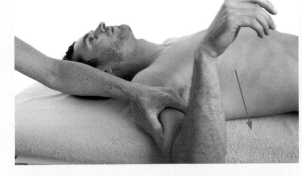

2) With the subject's elbow flexed and supinated, gently apply a CTM lock across the bicipital aponeurosis; ask him to extend and/or pronate the elbow.

3) With the elbow flexed, apply a lock deep to the biceps brachii for the brachialis; ask the subject to extend his elbow.

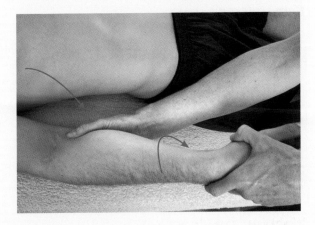

STR to the brachioradialis in supine:

1) With the subject's elbow flexed and the thumb facing upwards, grasp either side of the brachioradialis; ask him to extend his elbow while keeping his thumb facing up. Lock into the muscle itself and perform the same movement.

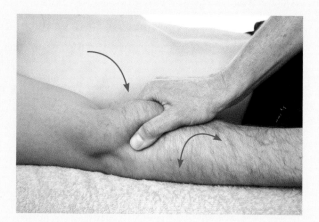

2) With the elbow in a supinated position, lock into the muscle and ask the subject to pronate his elbow. With the elbow in pronated position, lock in and ask him to supinate his elbow.

- This can be done with the elbow flexed or extended, depending on the resting tone of the muscle (flexing the elbow will shorten the fibres). Try combining elbow extension with supination and pronation.

STR to the triceps brachii in prone:

1) With the shoulder and elbow at 90 degrees, grasp either side of the triceps; ask the subject to flex his elbow. Use a reinforced thumb to lock in away from the olecranon process; ask him to flex his elbow.

STR to the triceps brachii in supine:

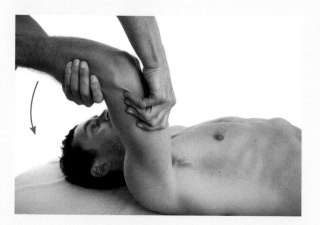

1) Hold the elbow and extend the shoulder to 180 degrees. With the other hand, grasp either side of the triceps and flex the elbow.

2) Still supporting the elbow, ask the subject to extend his elbow himself; grasp either side of the triceps and ask him to flex his elbow. Lock into the belly of the muscle and ask him to flex his elbow.

3) Lock into the tendon of the long head by applying pressure through the posterior deltoid towards the infraglenoid tubercle of the scapula; ask the subject to flex his elbow.

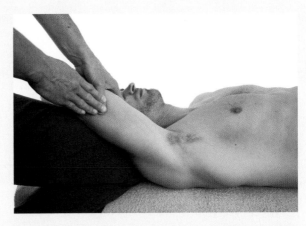

- To help release the long head of the triceps, apply a lock and ask the subject to flex or abduct his shoulder.

4) Use reinforced thumbs to apply a CTM lock away from the olecranon process; ask him to flex his elbow.

STR to the anconeus in supine:

1) Apply a CTM lock away from the lateral epicondyle of the humerus to address the origin of the anconeus; ask the subject to flex his elbow. Apply a CTM lock away from the olecranon process and ulna and ask the subject to flex his elbow.

STR to the supinator in supine:

1) With the elbow extended and supinated, lock into the supinator with fingers towards the lateral epicondyle; ask the subject to slowly pronate his forearm.

STR to the pronator teres in supine:

1) With the elbow flexed and in pronation, lock into the pronator teres directly palpable in between the brachioradialis and the forearm flexors; ask the subject to supinate his elbow. Apply a lock towards the radius attachment.

- Lock in, and extend and supinate the elbow for a greater stretch.

STR to the pronator quadratus in supine:

1) With the elbow in pronation, use fingers to lock in deep to the wrist flexors, away from the radius and towards the ulna; ask the subject to supinate his forearm.

The Forearm, Wrist and Hand

4

In the upper limb there are muscles common to the elbow, forearm, wrist, hand and fingers, and as mentioned earlier for the elbow, these muscles must be examined in a clinical setting as part of that chain. Restriction of a common muscle may have a completely different effect on hand and finger movement when compared to the wrist.

Of the forearm muscles, only the supinator and pronator teres have a primary function at the elbow, the remainder acting mainly on the wrist and hand. These are the extrinsic muscles of the hand and work in combination with the smaller intrinsic muscles. In this book only the action and effect of restriction of extrinsic muscles will be discussed (note that sometimes the term 'hand' will be used and at other times, 'wrist' or 'fingers', depending on the context of the discussion).

The wrist joint is formed by the distal end of the ulna and radius of the forearm and two rows of carpal bones. The hand consists of phalangeal bones. In total there are 28 bones in the hand and wrist.

The joints comprise the distal radioulnar joint, and the radiocarpal, midcarpal and intercarpal joints. In the hand there are two carpometacarpal joints, with five intercarpal articulations and metacarpal phalangeal (MCP) joints, proximal interphalangeal (PIP) joints and distal interphalangeal (DIP) joints.

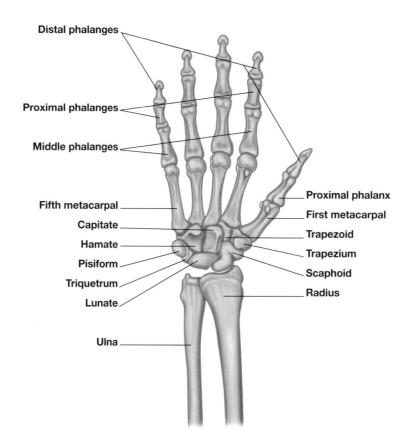

Figure 4.1: Structure of the wrist and hand.

Movement of the Wrist and Hand Joints

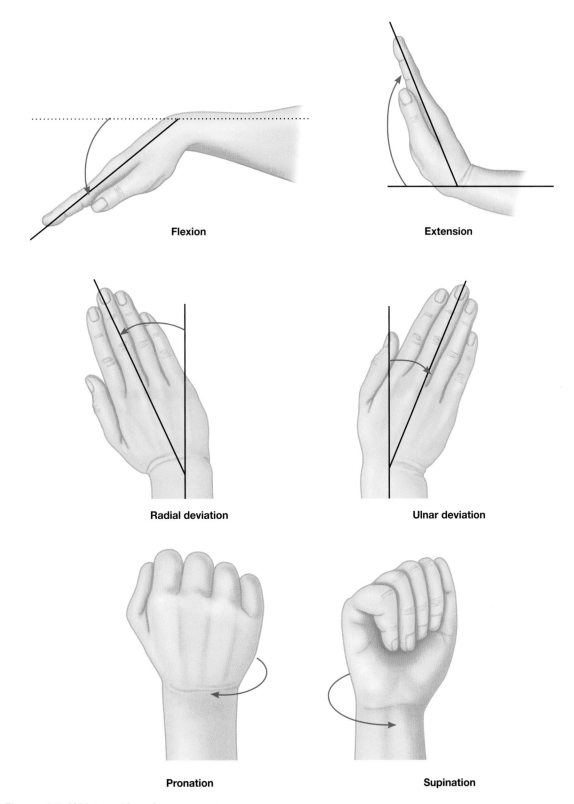

Figure 4.2: Wrist and hand movement.

The joints of the wrist and hand (fingers) are complex and only the essential gross (or osteokinematic) movements will be considered in this book. The wrist is the junction between the forearm and the hand. The gross motion of the wrist is measured in a clinical setting by observing the position of the hand as follows:

- Motion in the joints of the hand is observed by motion of the fingers and the thumb. Flexion of the fingers takes place at all of the joints (MCP, DIP, PIP), with limited extension. In humans the thumb has a unique movement whereby the pads of the thumb can be placed in contact with the pads of each finger. This is a combination of several movements known as opposition (Figure 4.3).

- Flexion and extension of the fingers results from a combination of extrinsic and intrinsic muscle action of the hand in a complex and coordinated manner, with each muscle taking the role of agonist, antagonist and stabiliser, depending on which finger is required to move.

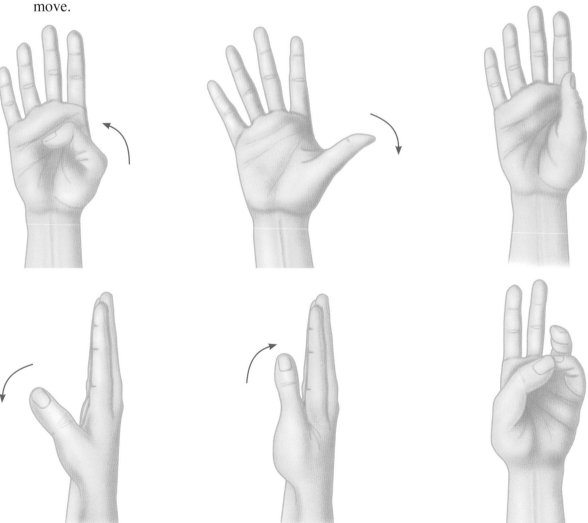

Figure 4.3: Opposition of the thumb.

Muscles of the Forearm, Wrist and Hand

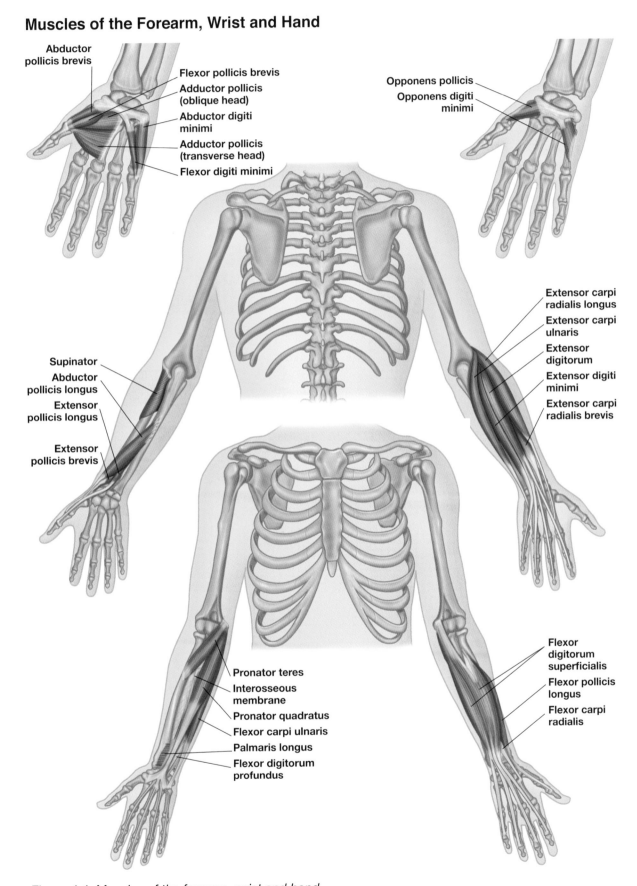

Figure 4.4: Muscles of the forearm, wrist and hand.

Muscle	Movement of the forearm, hand, fingers and thumb						
	Flexion	Extension	Supination	Pronation	Abduction	Adduction	Rotation
Pronator teres	F			F			
Flexor carpi radialis	H				H		
Palmaris longus	H						
Flexor carpi ulnaris	H				H		
Flexor digitorum superficialis	P						
Flexor digitorum profundus	P						
Flexor pollicis longus	T						
Pronator quadratus				F H			
Extensor carpi radialis (brevis and longus)		H			H		
Extensor digitorum		P H					
Extensor digiti minimi		Fifth P					
Extensor carpi ulnaris		H				H	
Supinator			F				
Abductor pollicis longus		T			T H		T
Abductor pollicis brevis					T		T
Adductor pollicis	T					T	
Flexor pollicis brevis	T				T		T
Opponens pollicis	T				T		T
Extensor pollicis brevis		T			H		
Extensor pollicis longus		T					

Key				F	H	P	T
	Primary role	Secondary role	Possible role	Forearm	Hand	Fingers	Thumb

Table 4.1: Movement of the forearm, hand, fingers and thumb.

Isolated restriction of the forearm, wrist and hand muscles is uncommon. Table 4.2 summarises the possible effects of restrictions in some of these muscles.

Muscle	Effect of tightness/restriction
Pronator quadratus and teres	Forearm held in position of increased pronation, with decreased or difficult supination. This is less pronounced with the elbow flexed because of the shortening of the teres.
Flexor carpi radialis	Wrist flexion towards radial side.
Flexor carpi ulnaris	Wrist flexion towards the ulnar side.
Flexor digitorum superficialis	Flexion contracture of middle phalanges.
Flexor digitorum profundus	Claw deformity, but usually in combination with other muscle issues.
Extensor carpi radialis (brevis and longus)	Decreased flexion and ulnar deviation, which has an impact on many activities of daily living.
Extensor digitorum	Hyperextension deformity of metacarpophalangeal joints.
Supinator	Elbow flexion with forearm supination, affecting pronation-supination movement.
Adductor pollicis	Adduction deformity of thumb, having implications for pinch and grasp, with considerable functional impairment.

Table 4.2: Effects of muscle restrictions on wrist and hand movement.

Effects of Forearm Muscle Tightness in Sport and Everyday Life

Climbing

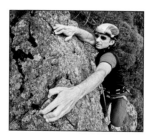

Climbing activities place considerable stress on the wrist and hand joints, and specifically on the forearm muscles. EMG studies demonstrate that the flexor digitorum superficialis and profundus are key muscles in many climbing grips and are consequently prone to injury. Any restriction in this muscle is therefore likely to lead to early fatigue, an inability to form a proper grip or muscle injury.

Squash

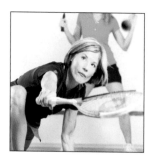

In the squash forehand drive, the wrist moves rapidly from a position of extension and supination to one of flexion and pronation. Studies of squash players have shown that hand flexion at the wrist joint and pronation of the forearm at the radioulnar joint contribute 30% of the segmental rotation required to achieve a fast forehand drive. Any restriction of the wrist extensors or flexors will limit the ability and speed of the necessary wrist movement and potentially lead to 'tennis elbow' or 'squash elbow'.

Typing

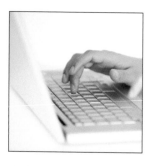

Using a keyboard or mouse for long periods while working on a computer is common. In the long term the wrist may be held in slight extension, thus shortening the wrist extensors, while at the same time the finger flexors are shortened. This combination can potentially lead to contracture of the fingers and a weakened grip, as well as compression at the wrist and an increased chance of carpal tunnel syndrome.

Soft Tissue Release to the Wrist and Hand

The multitude of different muscles working together to provide strength for gripping, as well as offering a range of precise movements, can be difficult to isolate. Make a note of the subject's passive and active ROM. Use active wrist and digit movement to help decipher which muscle groups are being addressed and always consider their secondary movements. Ensure that both flexor and extensor retinaculums are addressed, as tendons can become adhered to them and also some tendons originate from the retinaculums. Consider the interosseous membrane, since it is also an important attachment site.

STR to the wrist flexors (superficial compartment – flexor carpi ulnaris, palmaris longus, flexor carpi radialis, middle and deep layer – flexor digitorum superficialis, flexor digitorum profundus and flexor pollicis longus) in supine:

1) With the elbow supinated and semi-flexed, gently grasp the forearm with one hand on the extensor side. Use a soft fist of the other hand to apply a broad surface lock away from the wrist into the flexors; ask the subject to extend his wrist. For a more specific lock use a phalange, reinforced with the thumb, or use a knuckle for deeper work.

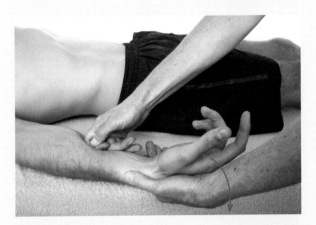 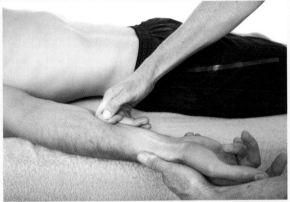

2) With the elbow supinated, position the arm on the couch, with the wrist off the side of the couch. Use fingers or knuckles to apply deeper locks. Use reinforced thumb or finger pressure to apply CTM locks between the different flexor muscles. Ask the subject to extend his wrist.

- Try a CTM lock at the common flexor tendon.

STR to the wrist extensors (extensor carpi radialis longus, extensor carpi radialis brevis, extensor carpi ulnaris, extensor digitorum communis, extensor indicis, extensor digiti minimi, extensor pollicis longus and extensor pollicis brevis) in supine:

1) With the elbow pronated and semi-flexed, gently grasp the forearm with one hand on the flexor side. Use a soft fist of the other hand to apply a broad surface lock away from the wrist into the extensors; ask the subject to flex his wrist.

2) With the elbow pronated, position the arm on the couch, with the wrist off the side of the couch; this will allow for a greater stretch. Use fingers or knuckles to apply deeper locks. Use reinforced thumb or finger pressure to apply CTM locks between the different extensor muscles.

3) Use reinforced thumbs to address the common extensor tendon with a CTM lock; ask the subject to flex his wrist.

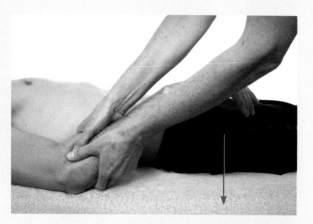

- If there is a chronic tendinopathy at the common extensor tendon, be careful not to overtreat; apply any lock cautiously, and if the tendon is particularly inflamed, avoid that spot altogether

4) Support the wrist with both hands and use thumbs to lock into the extensor tendons at the wrist. Apply locks in between the tendons and the extensor retinaculum; gently flex the wrist.

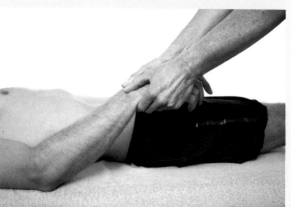

- Try combining with wrist abduction (check the next section). When isolating the extensor carpi ulnaris, close to the ulnar shaft, try asking the subject to abduct his wrist for the stretch.

STR to the wrist abductors (flexor carpi radialis, extensor carpi radialis longus, extensor carpi radialis brevis, abductor pollicis longus and extensor pollicis brevis) in supine:

1) With the elbow flexed, use a knuckle or a reinforced thumb to apply a lock; guide the subject into wrist adduction.

2) With the elbow supinated, position the arm on the couch, with the wrist off the side of the couch. Gently hook fingers behind the lateral epicondyle; ask the subject to adduct his wrist.

STR to the wrist adductors (flexor carpi ulnaris and extensor carpi ulnaris) in supine:

1) With the elbow extended, use a reinforced thumb to apply a CTM lock across the common flexor tendon; ask the subject to abduct his wrist. Apply a lock in the belly of the muscle and apply a CTM lock away from the pisiform; ask him to abduct his wrist.

STR to the thumb flexors (flexor pollicis brevis, opponens pollicis and flexor pollicis longus) in supine:

1) Lock into the thenar eminence to locate the pollicis flexor muscles; ask him to extend his thumb. Locate the flexor pollicis longus in the forearm and ask him to extend his thumb and wrist.

STR to the thumb extensors (extensor pollicis longus, extensor pollicis brevis and abductor pollicis longus) in supine:

1) Lock into the tendons of the thumb and flex the joints. Lock into the tendons on either side of the 'anatomical snuff box'; ask the subject to flex his thumb.

STR to the thumb abductors (abductor pollicis longus and abductor pollicis brevis) in supine:

1) Lock into the tendons, flex and adduct the joints.

STR to the thumb opposition muscles (opponens pollicis and flexor pollicis brevis) in supine:

1) Ask the subject to oppose his thumb by touching it with the fifth finger. Apply a lock into the thenar eminence; ask the subject to open out his hand.

STR to the thumb adductors (adductor pollicis) in supine:

1) Ask the subject to abduct his thumb by touching it with his index finger. Use a finger and thumb to gently pinch into the webbing at the base of the thumb; ask the subject to open his hand (abduct his thumb).

STR to the finger flexors (flexor digitorum superficialis, flexor digitorum profundus, flexor pollicis longus, flexor digiti minimi brevis lumbricals and interossei) in supine:

1) Apply CTM locks close to each metacarpophalangeal joint; ask the subject to extend his fingers.

STR to the finger extensors (extensor digitorum communis, extensor indicis, extensor digiti minimi, extensor pollicis longus and extensor pollicis brevis) in supine:

1) Apply CTM locks between the metacarpals on the dorsal surface of the hand; ask the subject to flex his fingers.

STR to the hand abductors (dorsal interossei, abductor digiti minimi and abductor pollicis brevis) in supine:

1) With the hand open, use a reinforced thumb to lock into points on the dorsal side of the hand; ask the subject to adduct his fingers. Combine this movement with wrist flexion to increase the stretch.

2) With the hand open and the fingers slightly flexed, lock into the hypothenar eminence; ask him to adduct his little finger.

STR to the hand adductors (palmar interossei and adductor pollicis) in supine:

1) Use a reinforced thumb to lock into points on the palmar side of the hand; ask the subject to abduct his fingers. Combine this movement with wrist extension to increase the stretch.

The Torso: Thoracic and Lumbosacral Spine

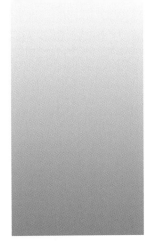

5

In this book the torso includes the part of the body encompassing the thoracic and lumbosacral spine, rib cage and abdominals. Inevitably some of the larger muscles cross or have an impact on the torso. These will only be covered in so much as when they directly affect the torso; otherwise they will be discussed in their primary sections. For example, the latissimus dorsi is covered in the shoulder girdle section.

For convenience, the torso is divided into the thoracic spine and the lumbosacral spine. The lumbosacral section includes the lumbar and sacral spine with the sacroiliac joints and lumbosacral movements.

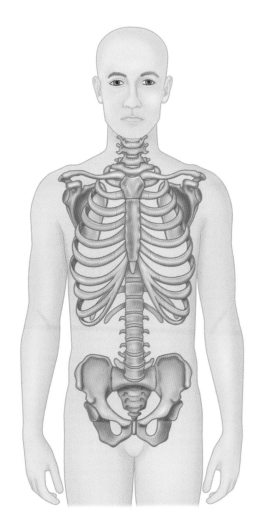

Figure 5.1: The torso.

Thoracic Spine

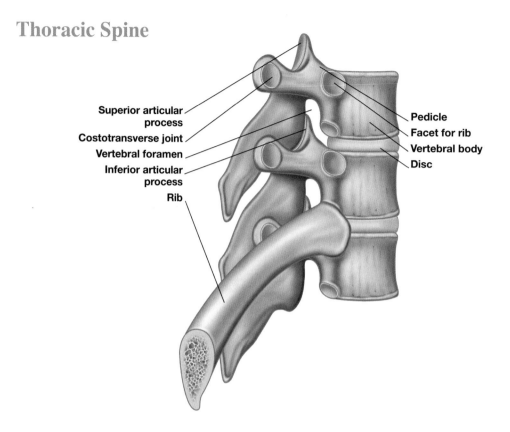

Superior articular
process
Costotransverse joint
Vertebral foramen
Inferior articular
process
Rib

Pedicle
Facet for rib
Vertebral body
Disc

Figure 5.2: Thoracic spine segment.

Movements of Thoracic Spine

The combination of the lowest ratio of disc to vertebral body height, facet joint orientation and rib attachments makes the thoracic spine the least mobile of the spinal sections. Like the cervical spine, it has osteokinematic movements as observed by torso or body movements (Figure 5.3), as well as arthrokinematic and coupled motions taking place at individual articulations.

Gross Observational Movements

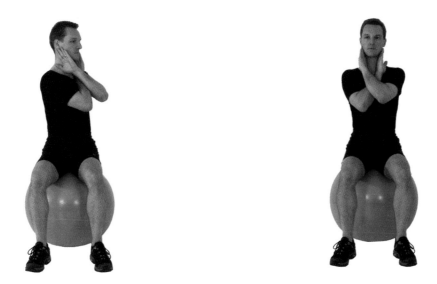

Figure 5.3: Osteokinematic thoracic rotation.

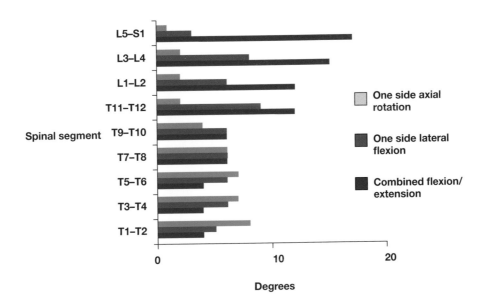

Figure 5.4: Thoracic and lumbar segmental motion.

The facet joint orientation largely determines the motion available at each segmental level. Working down the thoracic spine, the thoracic facet joints become more vertical and aligned to the frontal plane; this increases the potential for rotation and flexion.

Rib Cage Motion

A discussion of the motion of the thoracic spine would not be complete without mentioning movement of the rib cage. The ribs connect to the thoracic vertebrae by synovial joints on the vertebral body and the transverse processes, and then all but the last two extend around to connect at the front via costal cartilages and the sternum.

The key motions of the rib cage associated with breathing are termed 'pump action' and 'bucket handle', both of which are hinge-type motions. Bucket handle motion represents movement in the frontal plane, whereas pump action motion is in the sagittal plane.

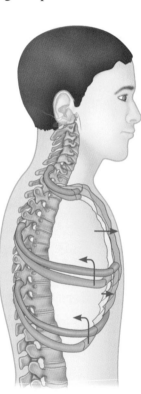

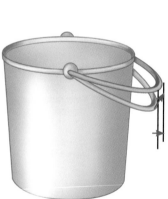

Figure 5.5: Rib motion.

Lumbosacral Spine

The lumbosacral spine comprises five lumbar vertebrae and five fused sacral vertebrae; its lower end joins the coccyx, the final segment of the vertebral column.

The sacroiliac joints are synovial joints formed between the auricular surfaces of the sacrum and the ilium. Much of the movement seen as lumbar spine movement is actually lumbosacral movement, or lumbar movement affected by sacroiliac movement.

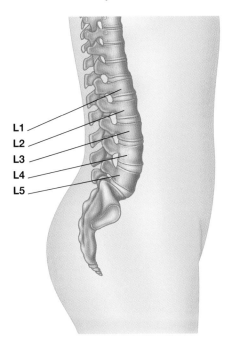

Figure 5.6: Lumbar spine.

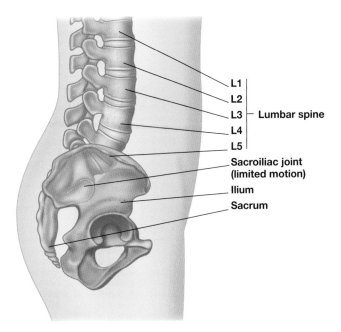

Figure 5.7: Sacroiliac joint.

Movements of the Lumbar Spine

Gross, or osteokinematic, movements of the lumbar spine are flexion, extension, lateral bending and rotation. The amount at each segment can be seen in Figure 5.4. As with all the sections of the spine, motion is determined to a great extent by the orientation of the facet joints. In the lumbar spine the facets are orientated vertically, parallel to the sagittal plane, which favours flexion and extension but restricts rotation. This is aided by the increased ratio of disc to vertebral body height in the lumbar spine compared to the thoracic spine.

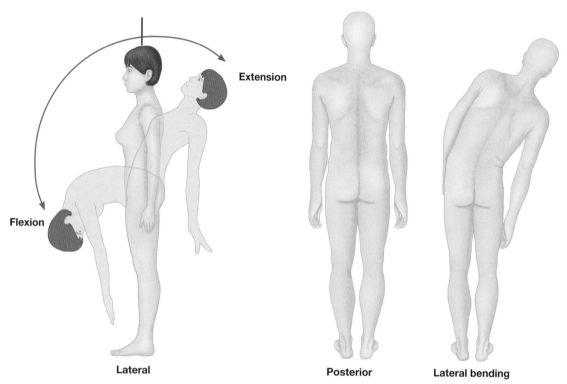

Figure 5.8: Range of motion of the lumbar spine.

Coupled Motion in the Thoracic and Lumbar Spine

In common with the cervical spine, the thoracic and lumbar spines exhibit coupled motion; however, in the thoracic it is not as consistent as in the cervical spine. The upper thoracic spine tends to link lateral flexion with ipsilateral rotation as in the lower cervical spine. Further down, the coupling is less consistent, with lateral flexion coupled with ipsilateral and contralateral flexion.

The lumbar spine exhibits small but essential coupled movements at the articular surfaces. Lumbar lordosis is considered to be the neutral position, and, although rotation is limited, side flexion and rotation are interdependent. Flexing or extending the lumbar spine will reduce the ability to rotate or laterally flex, and changes their relationship. In the neutral position, lateral flexion occurs with rotation to the contralateral side, whereas with lumbar flexion, rotation and lateral flexion occur in the same direction. Soft tissues – including muscles, ligaments and joint capsules – affect all of these movements, but particularly flexion. Extension is limited by the design of the facet joints and the spinous processes of adjacent vertebrae impacting on each other.

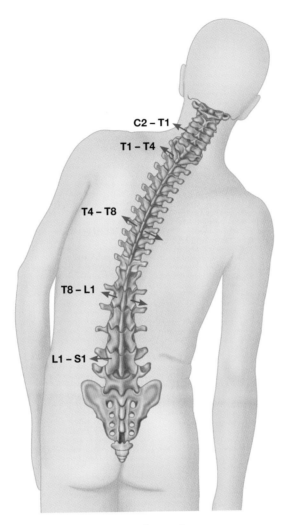

Figure 5.9: Coupled motion of the thoracic and lumbar spines.

Coordinated Lumbosacral Motion

One of the movements often seen as a measure of lumbar flexibility is the ability to touch the toes. However, this is actually a measure of the total lumbopelvic rhythm as determined by the motion of the sacroiliac joints and the lumbar spine. Initially the lumbar spine loses its lordosis and then the body pivots at the hip joints, with a small but essential movement occurring at the sacroiliac joints. This is a form of coupled motion and can be easily disrupted by restrictions not only in a number of soft tissues in the lumbar spine, but also in the gluteal and hamstring muscles.

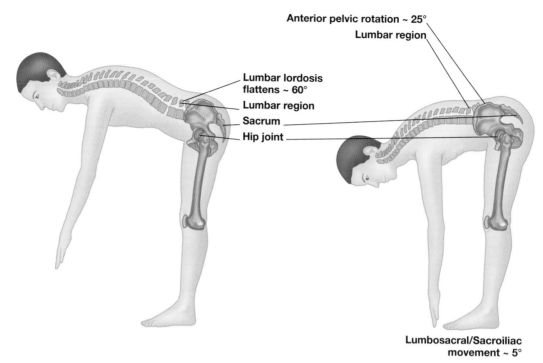

Figure 5.10: Lumbopelvic rhythm.

Thoracic and Lumbar Spine Muscles

Muscles affecting the lumbar and thoracic spines or the thorax also include muscles of the shoulder, abdomen and pelvis, as well as many smaller intrinsic muscles of the rib cage and lumbar spine. In this section, unless otherwise stated, only those muscles that have a specific functional role in thoracic or lumbar movement and are also capable of being directly affected by STR will be covered.

Muscles of the Thoracic and Lumbar Spines

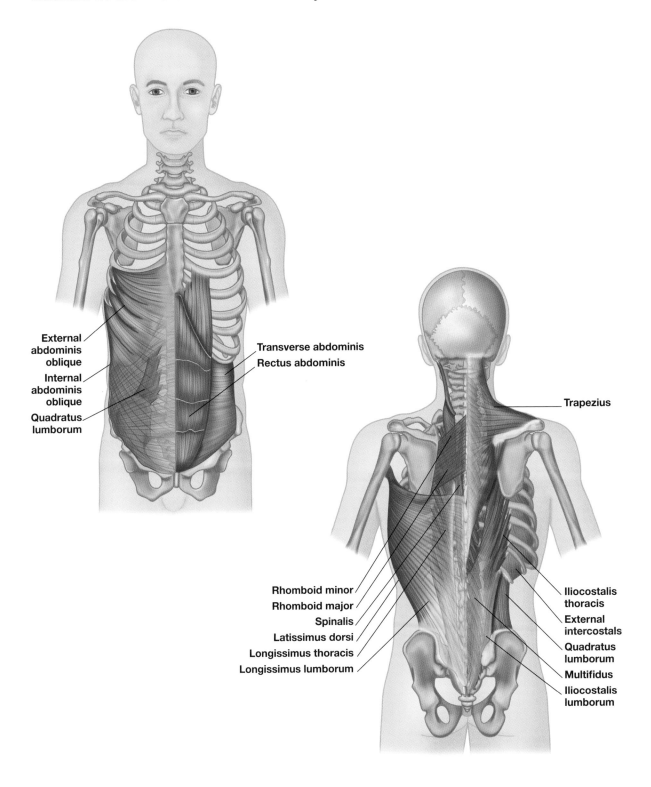

Figure 5.11: Muscles of the thoracic and lumbar spines.

Muscle	Movement of the thoracic and lumbosacral spines			
	Lateral flexion	Flexion	Extension	Rotation
Thoracic				
Spinalis	U		B	I-U
Longissimus thoracis pars thoracis	U		B	I-U
External intercostals				C
Lumbar				
Iliocostalis lumborum			B	I-U
Longissimus thoracis pars lumborum			B	I-U
Thoracolumbar				
Multifidus				C
Quadratus lumborum				
Internal obliques	U			I-U
External obliques	U			C-U
Rectus abdominis				
Other				
Latissimus dorsi	U	B		
Trapezius and rhomboids	U			C-U

Key				B	U	C	I
	Primary role	Secondary or weak role	Possible role	Bilateral	Unilateral	Contralateral	Ipsilateral

Table 5.1: Muscle movement at the thoracic and lumbosacral spines.

The relationship between the thoracic spine and the lumbosacral spine is such that tightness or restriction of one muscle is likely to have an effect on more than one section.

Muscle	Effect of tightness/restriction
Thoracic	
Spinalis	Postural deviations of upper torso, particularly lateral flexion and minor posterior rotation. Restricted upper body movement, especially flexion and contralateral rotation at segmental levels. Scoliosis.
Longissimus thoracis pars thoracis	Stiff thoracic region and reduced flexion in thoracic spine. Could contribute to overall reduction in lumbopelvic rhythm, with link to lumbar longissimus.
External intercostals	Increased difficulty with inspiration and decreased 'bucket handle' rib motion.
Lumbar	
Iliocostalis lumborum	Increased lumbar lordosis when in neutral stance, with reduced contralateral side bending.
Longissimus thoracis pars lumborum	Could impact on lumbopelvic rhythm and reduce ease of lumbar flexion.
Thoracolumbar	
Multifidus	Localised decreased contralateral lumbar side flexion and rotation. Reduction in lumbopelvic rhythm.
Quadratus lumborum	Increased ipsilateral flexion in neutral position. Reduction in lumbopelvic rhythm. Changes in gait. Perception of short leg on tight side with supine leg-length assessment.
Internal obliques	Limitations on contralateral posterior torso rotation and side flexion.
External obliques	Reduction in ipsilateral posterior torso rotation.
Rectus abdominis	Increased thoracolumbar flexion. Concomitant reduction in ease of inspiration and thoracolumbar extension.
Other	
Latissimus dorsi	Increased kyphotic posture.
Trapezius and rhomboids	Mid-upper thoracic spine ipsilateral rotation.

Table 5.2: Effects of muscle restrictions on thoracic and lumbosacral spine movement.

Effects of Thoracic and Lumbosacral Restrictions in Sport and Everyday Life

Hockey

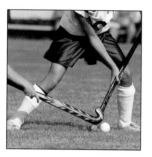

The requirement for considerable one-sided posture when playing hockey can lead to restrictions occurring in the quadratus lumborum (QL) and in the internal and external obliques. A forward-flexed position can result in a shortened rectus abdominis. Without regular stretching, the ability to change position when controlling the ball and to generate torque to provide hitting power may be impaired.

High Jump

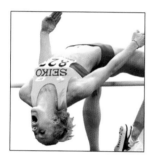

Generally in high jump the Fosbury flop technique is used, which requires a curved run-up and a rapid rotation of the body as the bar is cleared. Although much of this comes from using the limbs, a good jump requires strength, flexibility and stability in the obliques, abdominals and erector spinae muscles. The initial jump also requires powerful hamstrings, which will affect the lumbopelvic rhythm and the ability to extend the leg. Tightness in any of these areas will reduce performance.

Bending Over

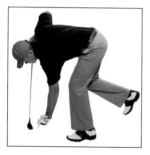

An everyday activity, taken for granted until a problem arises, bending over can be severely affected by tightness in lumbar and thoracic soft tissues. Tight hamstrings can stop normal lumbopelvic rhythm and force the abdominals to contract harder, potentially leading to long-term tightness. Tight erector spinae muscles, both lumbar and thoracic, can prevent the normal motion and increase the need for excessive hip flexion, resulting in greater compression on the lumbar spine. In the long term this will inhibit simple activities, including sitting down on a chair and getting up again.

Soft Tissue Release to the Spine and Thorax

Make a note of the subject's natural standing position. Check ROM: flexion, extension, rotation, and side flexion of the spine. Avoid treatment in the prone position, in which the subject may be susceptible to locking up his facet joints, for example if the vertebral discs are compressed or the lumbar spine has reduced lordosis. The side lying and seated positions are excellent for treating and opening up the lumbar spine in a functional way, whereby movements can be minimal and as specific as necessary to regain correct movement in particular segments of the spine.

Treat systematically and consider the attachment points and muscle borders, even if it is difficult to differentiate between muscles, such as the different branches of the erector spinae. Always consider the layering of different muscle groups as pressure is acquired. The transversospinales are the deepest intrinsic layer: as well as producing movement, they are vital in maintaining posture. Consideration of these particular muscles will help them to be targeted during strengthening programmes.

STR to the erector spinae (spinalis, longissimus and iliocostalis) in prone:

1) For the lumbar spine region, use a broad surface lock, such as a fist, to lock in on either side of the spine; guide the subject into a posterior pelvic tilt.

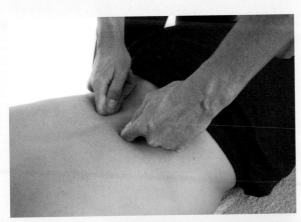
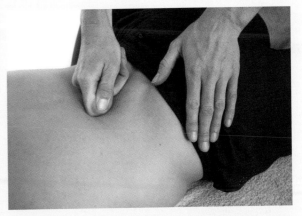

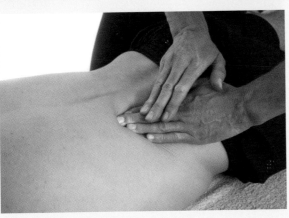

2) Progress to a deeper lock with the olecranon process, a phalange reinforced with the thumb or a knuckle; address the spinalis close to the spine in the lamina groove, the longissimus in the mid-line and the iliocostalis on the lateral line of the erector spinae 'bulk'. Guide the subject into a posterior pelvic tilt. Use fingers to curl around the lateral border of iliocostalis; guide the subject into a posterior pelvic tilt.

- In the lumbar region use CTM locks to specifically affect the thoracolumbar fascia.

- Avoid any pressure on the spinous processes.

3) Use a knuckle to apply a CTM lock into the lumbosacral junction; guide the subject into a posterior pelvic tilt.

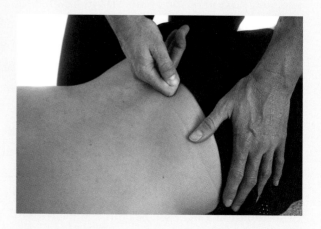

STR to the erector spinae in side lying:

1) Secure one hand on the subject's iliac crest and use a soft fist to lock in deep to the latissimus dorsi and into the superficial fibres of the erector spinae group; guide him into a posterior pelvic tilt.

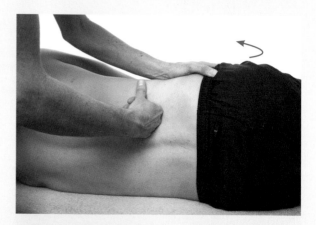

2) Progress to a deeper lock with the knuckle; address the spinalis in the lamina groove, the longissimus in the mid-line and the iliocostalis on the lateral line of the erector spinae 'bulk'. Guide the subject into a posterior pelvic tilt.

- Use a CTM lock as necessary to release the thoracolumbar fascia.

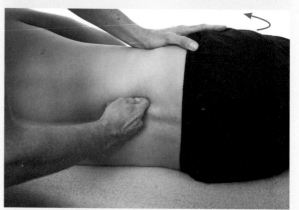

3) For the thoracic spinal area, lock in using a knuckle or reinforced thumb, again considering the three lines of muscle: spinalis in the lamina groove, the longissimus in the mid-line and the iliocostalis on the lateral line. Ask the subject to arch his back into the lock.

- Try curling around the iliocostalis with a CTM lock; avoid crushing tissues into the ribs.

- Between the scapulae, slowly drop the lock deep to the trapezius and rhomboids and feel the vertical direction of the erector spinae.

- Consider any presenting curvature of the spine when adding direction to the lock.

STR to the erector spinae in seated:

1) Ensure that the subject is stable, with his feet on the ground, and support his anterior shoulder gently. Use a soft fist to lock in; ask him to flex forwards or to side flex his spine.

2) Progress to using a knuckle to locate specific areas, for example close to the facet joints.

- Consider the direction of the lock, depending on his posture.

- Use a CTM lock and guide the subject in very precise, subtle movements to target his specific movement limitations.

STR to the transversospinales (multifidus, rotators, semispinalis) in prone:

1) Locate the multifidus in the lumbar spine. Use reinforced fingers or a thumb to lock in laterally away from the spinous processes; slowly move the erector spinae and increase the depth of the lock into the dense fibres of the multifidus. Ask the subject to perform a posterior pelvic tilt.

2) Use a CTM lock to directly engage the multifidus on the sacrum; guide the subject into a posterior pelvic tilt.

STR to the transversospinales (multifidus, rotators, semispinalis) in side lying:

1) Sacrum: use a CTM lock to directly engage the multifidus on the sacrum; guide the subject into a posterior pelvic tilt.

2) Lumbar spine: locate the multifidus on the lumbar spine. Use a knuckle to lock in laterally away from the spinous processes; slowly move the erector spinae as the depth of the lock is increased to reach the dense fibres of the multifidus. Ask the subject to perform a posterior pelvic tilt.

3) Thoracic spine: use a knuckle to slowly drop in to the lamina groove of the thoracic spine; ask the subject to slowly push back into the lock, by arching his back. Lock into the tissues in the same way and guide the subject into rotation to the same side.

- Try securing an elbow in your side to help attain a deep lock.

STR to the QL in side lying:

1) Position the subject in side lying, with a small pillow between his knees to help the pelvis into neutral. Use reinforced thumbs to slowly drop on to the lateral border of the QL; ensure that the lock is between the twelfth rib and the pelvis while being deep to the erector spinae group. Ask him to extend and adduct his hip (to depress his pelvis) and abduct his arm (to elevate the twelfth rib), thus providing a small stretch to the QL.

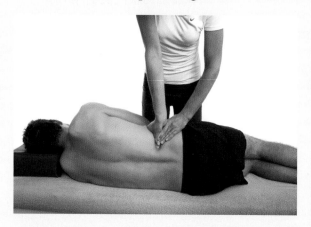 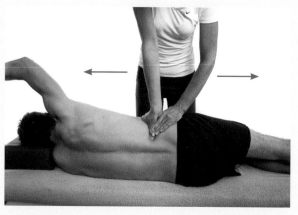

STR to the QL in seated:

1) Ensure that the subject's feet are firmly on the ground. Stand to his side and ask him to place his hands on his opposite knee. Use your thumb reinforced with your fingers to slowly target the lateral border of the QL as he exhales. Ask him to slowly flex towards his hands as he inhales; release the pressure as he uses his hands to push himself back up to the seated position.

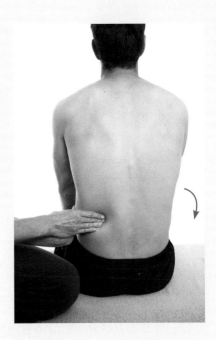

STR to the rectus abdominis in supine:

1) Place the subject in crook lying position and ask him to flex his trunk into a half sit-up. Use your fingers to lock on either side of the rectus abdominis lateral borders and direct the lock down towards the pubis. Ask him to extend back down onto the couch.

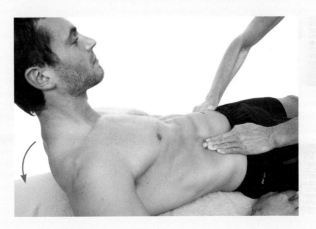

2) Use your fingers to apply a CTM lock close to the pubis and direct the lock laterally. Ask him to side flex his spine to the opposite side.

STR to the rectus abdominis in seated:

1) Stand behind the subject and ask him to flex his spine forwards a few degrees. Use fingers to apply a CTM lock by curling in and slightly under the muscle; ask the subject to extend his spine back and slowly hyperextend for an increased stretch.

   • Try locking in one side at a time and asking him to side flex his spine to the opposite side.

STR to the external and internal obliques in supine:

1) Place your cupped hand on the external oblique towards the lower eight ribs. Ask him to rotate his trunk to the opposite side; gently increase the hand pressure to a lock and ask him to rotate back down to the couch. Apply a lock away from the iliac crest and ask him to rotate back down to the couch.

- The direction of the lock will make all the difference with the efficacy of this release.

2) Lock into the internal oblique, with the fingers, towards the lower three ribs. Ask him to rotate his trunk to the opposite side. Lock in away from the linea alba and abdominal aponeurosis and away from the iliac crest; ask him to rotate his trunk to the opposite side.

STR to the external and internal obliques in seated:

1) Stand behind the subject. Lock in with both hands slightly cupped, one on each side, away from the lower ribs and towards the pubis; ask him to slowly extend his spine. Lock in away from the lower ribs and towards the iliac crest; ask him to extend his spine.

2) Stand to the side of the subject. Use one hand, with the thumb and index finger stretched apart, to lock in away from the lower ribs and towards the pelvis; ask him to side flex his spine to the other side.

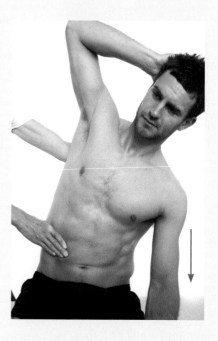

3) Use fingers to lock in away from the lower ribs and towards the pubis; ask him to rotate to the same side to stretch the external obliques. Lock in away from the ribs and towards the iliac crest; ask him to rotate to the opposite side for the internal oblique.

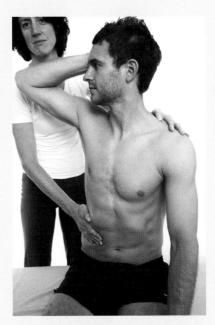 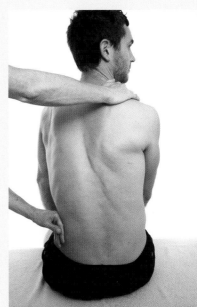

- Alter the direction of the lock according to how the fibres are lengthening and which oblique is being addressed.

STR to the diaphragm in supine:

1) Gently use fingers to hook in underneath the inferior edge of the rib cage, lateral to the xiphoid process, as the subject slowly inhales. Maintain this pressure and ask him to slowly exhale.

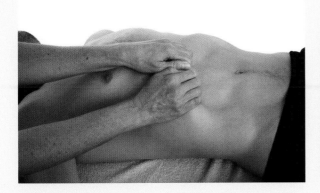 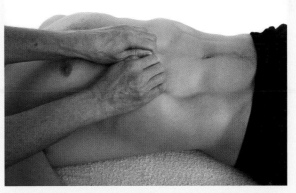

STR to the internal and external intercostals in supine:

1) Ensure that the muscles of the pectoralis major and minor and the serratus anterior have been warmed up. Use fingers to slowly apply a CTM lock into the first intercostal space, inferior to the clavicle and lateral to the sternum; ask the subject to slowly inhale and exhale. Move down one intercostal space at a time, locking and breathing.

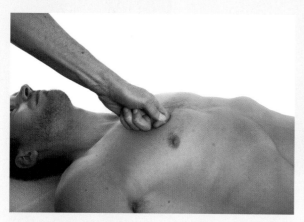 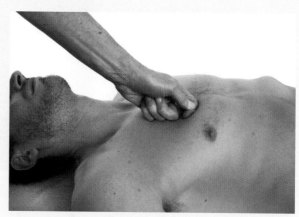

STR to the internal and external intercostals in side lying:

1) For the lateral intercostals the side lying position is easier. Use fingers to apply a CTM lock and ask him to inhale and exhale. Try locking deep to the external oblique, the serratus anterior and the latissimus dorsi.

- It is not possible to distinguish the internal from the external intercostals, except for the small anterior area where there are only internal intercostals, so maintain a lock as the subject inhales and exhales to target them both.

STR to the thoracolumbar fascia:

The thoracolumbar fascia is a broad, flat diamond-shaped tendon; it is thin but very dense. It lies superficially across the posterior thorax to the lower lumbar vertebrae, and extends across the sacrum to the posterior iliac crest. The most superficial layer lies superficial to the erector spinae, and the latissimus dorsi partially arises from it. The middle layer lies in between the erector spinae and the QL. The anterior and thinnest of the layers lies deep to the QL. All three layers converge together at the lateral border of the erector spinae and then extend across into the abdomen, forming the abdomen fascia; the transverse abdominis and internal oblique partially arise from it.

- The use of CTM locks when addressing the muscles that are anchored to the thoracolumbar fascia will provide effective release to the middle and lower spine and have body-wide consequences.

The Hip

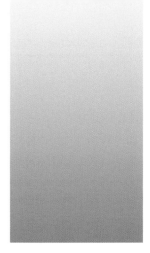

6

The hip joint is a synovial ball and socket joint. It is a very stable joint because it needs to resist the large forces generated when the lower limbs interact with the ground, and at the same time it has the necessary mobility for ambulation – the key task in everyday life as well as in almost all sporting activities. Forces into the hip joint can exceed, for example, seven times body weight in skiing and five times body weight in running.

Restrictions of the hip joint often occur through pathologies such as osteoarthritis. Like the glenohumeral (shoulder) joint, the hip joint has a capsule and labrum, which help provide stability and can contribute to restrictions. In this section, as in the rest of the book, we are simply concerned with the effect of muscle and associated soft tissue restrictions. However, pathologies like osteoarthritis are considered, in part, to be a result of abnormal forces and movement patterns at a joint surface.

ROM of the hip is also affected by the condition of the pelvis and lumbar spine. Thus, when completing a clinical assessment of hip joint restrictions, the ROM is usually measured in open chain, as a function of femur motion relative to the pelvis. In a practical environment a therapist will also examine movement patterns in closed-chain activities, to identify hip joint restrictions. This is particularly important when examining lumbopelvic rhythm (discussed in Chapter 5), in which the pelvis, low back and hip joints work in a synchronised fashion.

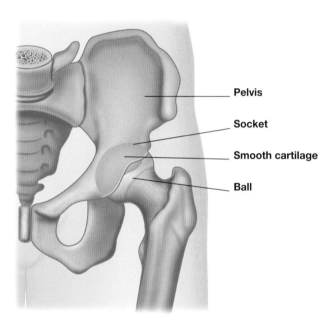

Figure 6.1: The hip joint.

Movement of the Hip Joint

Open-Chain ROM (Typical Clinical Assessment)

'Open chain' means that the distal joints/limbs (feet) are free to move. The alternative, 'closed chain', means the feet are fixed, normally as in weight bearing or when performing actions such as squatting. The closed-chain ROM of the hips is then dependent on other joints, including the ankles, knees and lumbar spine (see discussion of pelvis and lumbar spine in Chapter 5). The normal ranges for passive movement of the hip are given in Table 6.1.

Movement	Range (degrees)
Flexion	130
Extension	10
Abduction	45
Adduction	30
External rotation in flexion	40
External rotation in extension	40
Internal rotation in flexion	50
Internal rotation in extension	40

Table 6.1: Normal ranges for passive movement of the hip.

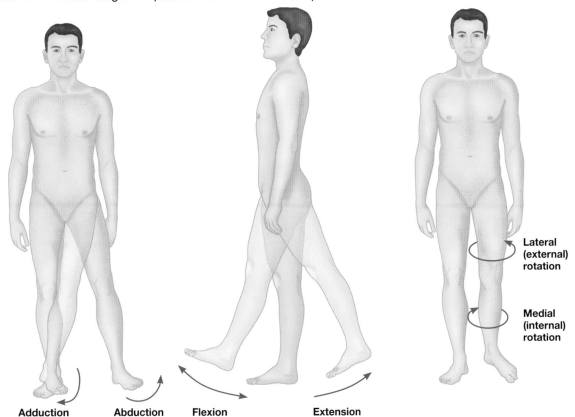

Figure 6.2: Hip joint range of motion.

Hip Joint Muscles

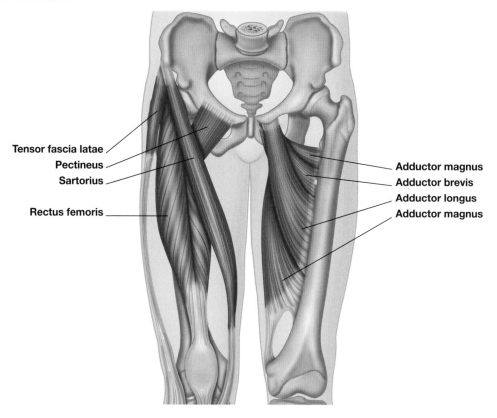

Tensor fascia latae

Pectineus

Sartorius

Rectus femoris

Adductor magnus

Adductor brevis

Adductor longus

Adductor magnus

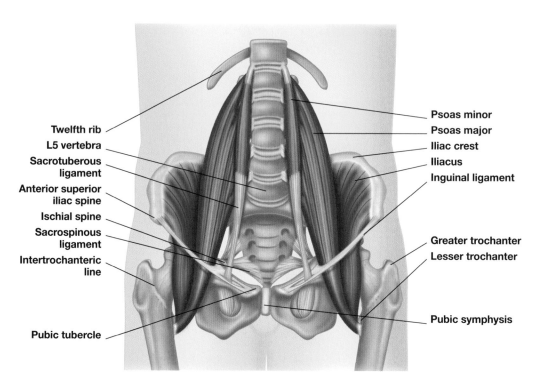

Twelfth rib

L5 vertebra

Sacrotuberous ligament

Anterior superior iliac spine

Ischial spine

Sacrospinous ligament

Intertrochanteric line

Pubic tubercle

Psoas minor

Psoas major

Iliac crest

Iliacus

Inguinal ligament

Greater trochanter

Lesser trochanter

Pubic symphysis

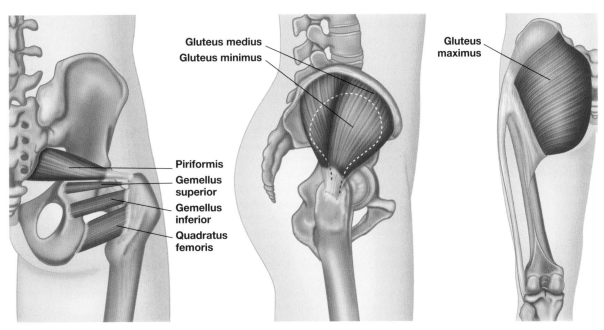

Figure 6.3: Hip joint muscles.

Muscle	Movement of the hip					
	Internal (medial) rotation	External (lateral) rotation	Flexion	Extension	Abduction	Adduction
Psoas major/minor	Possible	Possible	Primary			
Iliacus	Possible	Possible	Primary			
Gluteus maximus		Secondary		Primary		
Gluteus medius	Primary	Possible			Primary	
Gluteus minimus	Primary				Primary	
Pectineus			Possible			Primary
Adductor brevis	Possible					Primary
Adductor longus			Secondary			Primary
Adductor magnus				Secondary		Primary
Piriformis	Secondary	Primary				
Gemelli		Primary				
Quadratus femoris		Primary				
Obturator externus		Primary				
Rectus femoris		Secondary	Primary		Secondary	
Sartorius		Secondary	Primary		Secondary	
Tensor fasciae latae (TFL)	Primary		Primary		Secondary	

Key	Primary role	Secondary role	Possible role

Table 6.2: Muscle movement at the hip joint.

Muscle	Effect of tightness/restriction
Psoas	Reduced hip extension. Increased or sometimes decreased lumbar lordosis, depending on body position. Possible reduction in lateral flexion of trunk.
Iliacus	Reduced hip extension. Increased anterior pelvic tilt with compensatory increased lumbar lordosis.
Gluteus maximus	Limits hip flexion, medial rotation. Increased movement of lumbar spine in sporting activities.
Gluteus medius	Potential pelvic tilt to tight side. Reduced adduction.
Gluteus minimus	Potential pelvic tilt to tight side. Reduced adduction. Potential increased medial rotation.
Pectineus Adductor brevis Adductor longus Adductor magnus	Multitude of potential changes in gait, including scissor gait and reduced stride. Reduced hip abduction.
Piriformis Gemelli Quadratus femoris Obturator externus	Hard to detect individual restrictions, although piriformis restriction implicated with sciatica.
Rectus femoris	Limits hip extension in gait and may impact on lateral rotation (note the impact of muscle restriction with combined knee flexion and hip extension).
Sartorius	Possible reduction in hip extension.
Tensor fasciae latae (iliotibial band)	Potential to limit hip extension, adduction and lateral rotation of hip. (Note that these effects are more pronounced with knee motion.)

Table 6.3: Effects of muscle restrictions on hip joint movement.

Effects of Hip Restrictions in Sport and Everyday Life

Cycling

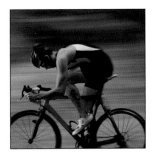

Cycling requires the use of all of the hip joint muscles, either working as prime movers or antagonist controllers. A restriction in the iliopsoas muscle will potentially increase low back pain and lead to compensatory shortening in leg extension or external rotation of the lower limb. Tightness in the tensor fasciae latae (TFL) can lead to a less efficient cycling style, as the hip, knee and ankle coordination is affected. In the long term this can also lead to trochanteric bursitis.

Skiing

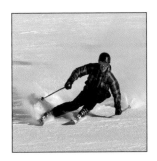

Almost all forms of competitive skiing require a high degree of hip mobility with strong stability. New ski technology has also made it easier for the recreational skier to indulge in carving skiing. This technique requires the turning ski hip to abduct and apply the turning force, whilst the uphill hip must adduct and flex to keep correct balance in the turn. Tightness in the glutes or iliotibial band (ITB) in the uphill hip will affect style, whilst tight adductors in the downhill leg will limit the ability to drop into the turn.

Sitting Down and Picking up Objects

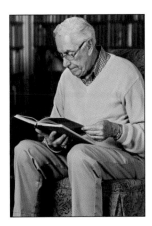

Hip flexion, essential for sitting down on low chairs or bending over to pick objects up, is restricted when the gluteal muscles are tight. This tightness will often cause increased flexion at the lumbar spine and potentially increase back pain when picking up objects. When sitting down on a low, soft chair, someone with tight gluteal muscles may find themselves dropping backwards into the chair, rather than using a controlled movement. It has also been shown that the normal lumbar lordosis is reduced with decreased thigh-trunk angle when in different seated postures, as a consequence of tight hip extensors, which is implicated in greater low back pain.

Soft Tissue Release to the Hip

Make a note of the subject's pelvis position when standing and when sitting. Check through hip ROM actively and passively.

STR to the psoas major and minor in supine:

1) Place the subject in crook lying position. Place fingers lateral to the rectus abdominis border at navel level. Gentle acquire pressure as the subject exhales. There are many layers of muscle tissue and fascia to feel through before the psoas. It may be possible to feel the psoas shorten on contraction (ask the subject to flex his hip). Once located, with the subject relaxed, ask him to slowly extend the hip, by straightening his leg, while keeping his heel on the couch.

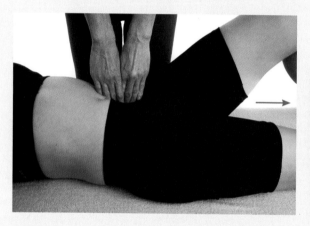 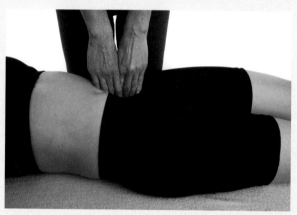

- Do not rush, and if the subject feels any pain across the abdomen it is important not to try to go any deeper. Often there may be restrictions, particularly in the fascia, higher up so it is important to treat at that level, rather than trying to force a deep pressure.

- If in doubt, avoid treating altogether and concentrate instead on the iliacus and the iliopsoas tendon.

STR to the iliacus in supine:

1) Place the subject in crook lying position. Start just lateral to the anterior superior iliac spine (ASIS) and slowly glide your fingers into the iliacus. Keep your fingers as close to the inside of the ilium as possible. Ask the subject to slowly extend his hip.

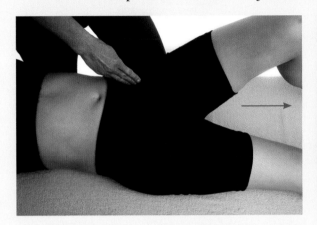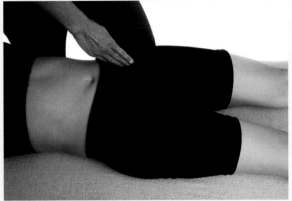

- If there is any restriction here, it may be possible to only hook over the crest of the ilium and not drop into the iliacus at all. Perform the stretch here. If STR is then performed on the opposite side, the original side will often have released by the time this is completed, so a deeper lock can be attained.

STR to the iliacus in side lying:

1) With the subject in side lying, gently curl the fingers into the iliacus. Ask the subject to extend his hip.

- Ensure that the pelvis stays in neutral during hip extension.

STR to the rectus femoris, sartorius and TFL in side lying:

1) Stand behind the subject and support his flexed knee with your arm. Use your fingers to direct a lock away from the ASIS into the sartorius origin. Extend the hip or ask him to extend for active STR. Ask him to extend his hip.

2) Use fingers to hook in and direct pressure away from the anterior inferior iliac spine (AIIS); ask him to extend the hip.

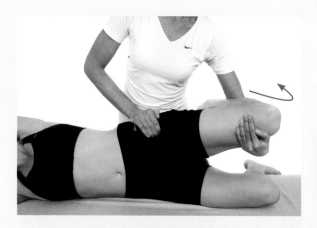
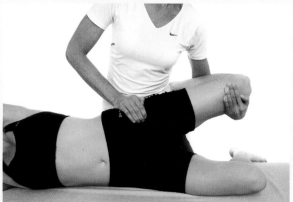

- This area may be ticklish or sensitive, so be decisive when acquiring the lock but do not rush.

- Ask the subject to do a posterior pelvic tilt for a more subtle stretch.

3) For the TFL, stand from behind and lock in with your elbow, clasping both hands together to guide the pressure. Ask the subject to extend his hip.

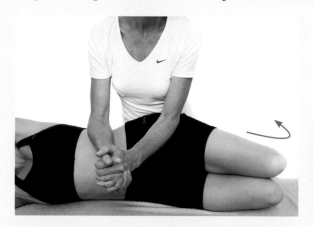
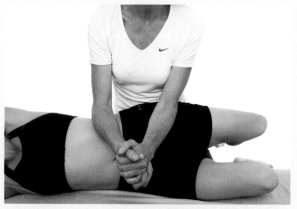

- The myofascia here is particularly dense so a CTM lock will provide a good release. Apply the pressure, maintain the depth and move the lock laterally towards you; ask the subject to lengthen.

STR to the rectus femoris, sartorius and TFL in supine:

1) Apply a lock in and down, away from the ASIS; lock inferiorly for the rectus femoris and sartorius, and laterally from the ASIS for the TFL. Direct the subject into a posterior pelvic tilt.

2) Use a reinforced thumb to apply a CTM lock across the tendon of the rectus femoris; ask him to straighten his leg out along the couch to extend his hip.

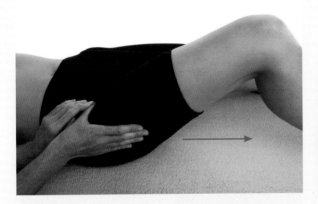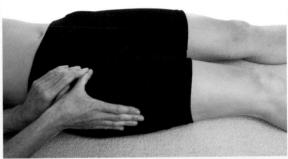

3) Stand on the opposite side of the couch and position a knee on the subject's nearside lateral hip. Lean across and hook fingers into his opposing TFL and pull a CTM lock gently from the lateral edge towards the medial edge. Ask the subject to laterally rotate his hip.

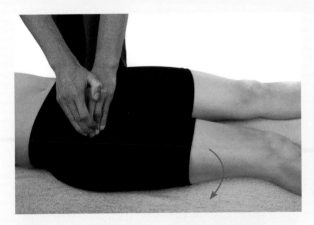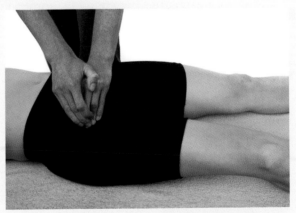

STR to the gluteus maximus in prone:

1) With the knee flexed to 90 degrees, gently grasp the ankle. Use the heel of a hand, a fist or an elbow to lock into the gluteus maximus; move the hip into medial rotation. Lock in away from the iliac crest, lock in away from the sacrum and lock into the belly of the muscle; slowly acquire a deeper pressure as the muscle relaxes. Move the hip into medial rotation.

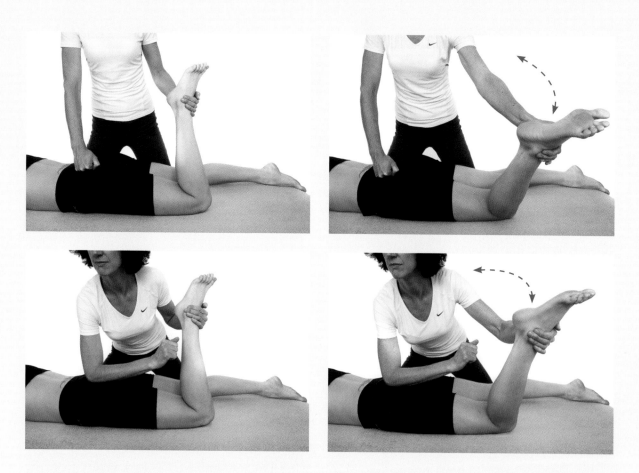

2) Passive STR is easy to perform and highly effective, but active STR is useful for particularly dense tissue; it is also beneficial for someone with reduced ROM (work within the comfortable range). Apply a lock and ask him to medially rotate his hip; it may be necessary to place a hand on his lateral ankle to guide him through the correct movement.

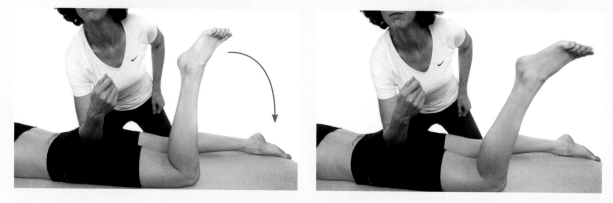

- Use a CTM lock at the iliac and sacrum attachments.

- Compare ROM in medial rotation on both sides before treatment.

- Avoid moving the leg too far as it may put stress on the medial knee. The pelvis should be maintained in neutral position.

STR to the gluteus maximus is side lying:

1) Position the subject on his side with both knees together and flexed. Apply a lock and ask him to flex his hip. Lock in away from the ilium; lock in away from the sacrum.

2) Use a reinforced thumb to curl under the gluteus maximus as it inserts into the gluteal line.

- This method of treatment links in well with STR performed to the lower back.

STR to the gluteus medius and minimus in prone:

1) With the knee flexed to 90 degrees, gently grasp the ankle. Use an elbow or a fist to lock into the gluteus medius. Move the hip into lateral rotation. Progress the lock deep through the gluteus medius to affect the gluteus minimus. To treat the posterior fibres of the gluteus medius, apply a lock and move the hip into medial rotation.

- CTM locks work well here, as the muscles are often inhibited and can have tight irritable fascia! A good release will enhance strengthening programmes.

STR to the gluteus medius and minimus and the TFL in side lying:

1) Position the subject on his side as far towards the end of the couch as possible. Pick up his flexed upper leg, supporting the knee, and abduct to shorten the muscles. Lock in using the heel of the hand or use two or three knuckles for a deeper lock; slowly drop the leg back down to adduct the hip.

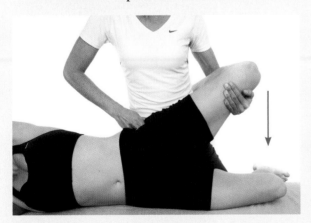
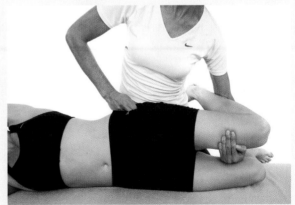

2) Position the subject on his side with both knees together and flexed. Ask him to lift his knee while keeping his ankles together. Apply a lock into the shortened gluteus medius and ask him to drop his knee slowly down, for hip adduction. Apply a deeper lock for the gluteus minimus.

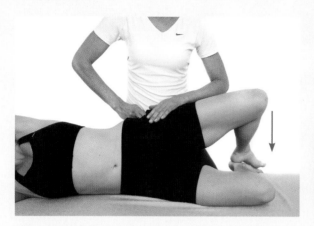 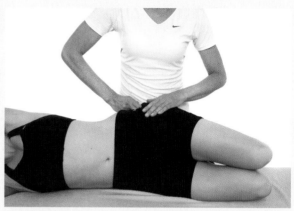

3) To treat the TFL, ask the subject to lift his knee while keeping his ankles together, and using your fingers or elbow, lock into the TFL; ask him to drop his knee back down for hip adduction or ask him to flex his hip.

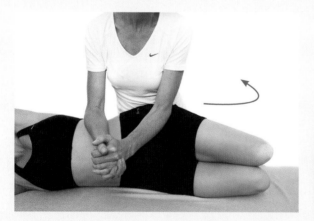 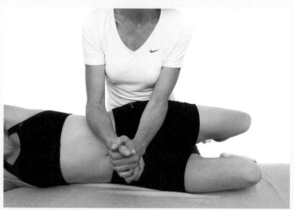

- A CTM lock will provide the most effective release here, as the fascia commonly becomes thickened because of the role these muscles play in stability and the fact that they run into the thick band of connective tissue: the ITB.

STR to the deep lateral rotators in prone:

1) Ensure that the gluteus maximus is relaxed and warmed up. With the knee flexed to 90 degrees, gently grasp the ankle. Use an elbow to slowly apply a deep pressure through the gluteus maximus into the belly of the piriformis (halfway between the middle of the sacrum and the greater trochanter). Maintain this pressure and move the hip into medial rotation.

2) With the knee flexed to 90 degrees, gently grasp the ankle. Use your fingers to locate the quadratus femoris (halfway between the greater trochanter and the ischial tuberosity). Move the hip into medial rotation.

- STR can be done actively, but people often find this difficult without a point of reference. Try placing your hand on the subject's lateral malleolus to guide the required movement.

STR to the deep lateral rotators in side lying:

1) Position the subject on his side with both knees together and flexed. Slowly apply a lock into the piriformis. Ask him to lift his ankle for medial rotation.

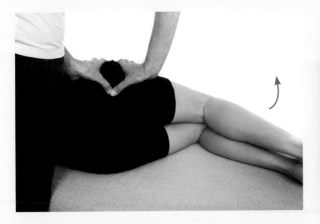 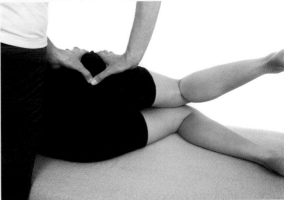

2) Lock in at points around the greater trochanter, each time asking the subject to lift his ankle. This will affect all of the lateral rotators; also lock in towards the pelvis and ischium.

- This can be very precise and easier to administer than in the prone position. It is also easier to perform active STR.

- Releasing the tissue around the greater trochanters has significant impact on the whole of the pelvis.

STR to the hamstrings in supine:

1) Position the subject with his hip flexed and his lower leg resting on your shoulder. Lock in away from the origin with fingers or with a thumb reinforced with fingers; slowly move his leg with your shoulder to flex his hip. Use a CTM lock at the origin of the hamstring.

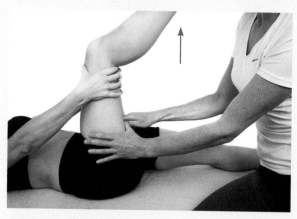 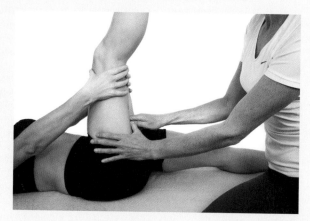

2) In the same position ask the subject to grasp behind his knee. Lock in away from the origin and ask him to pull his knee forwards to flex his hip.

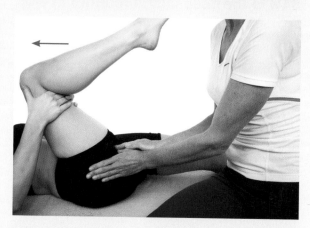

STR to the hamstrings in side lying:

1) Position the subject on his side with both knees together and flexed. Use fingers or a reinforced thumb to apply a CTM lock to the hamstring origin; ask the subject to flex his hip. Apply locks, away from the ischium, and ask him to flex his hip. For a greater stretch, ask him to flex his hip and extend his knee.

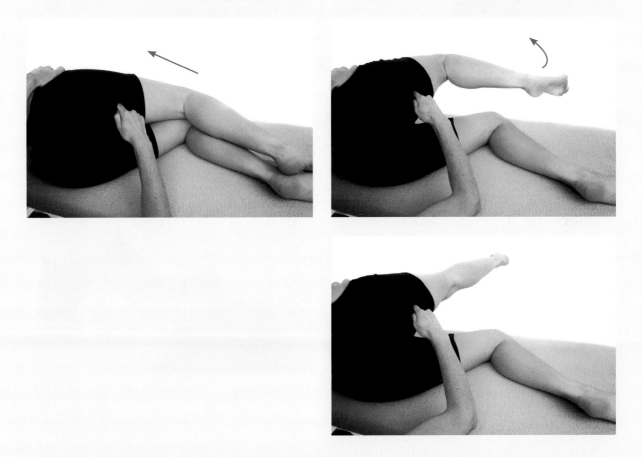

STR to the adductors in supine:

1) Sit on the couch, with subject's knee flexed and hip laterally rotated; support his knee with your hand and apply a lock away from the pubis. Either gently drop his knee for hip abduction or ask him to push his knee into your hand for active STR.

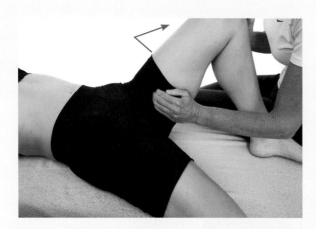
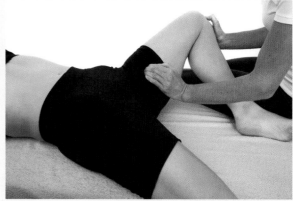

2) Position your leg under his knee and apply a CTM lock close to the origin; ask the subject to abduct into your leg.

3) Position the subject in supine at the end of the couch; with the subject's knee flexed over the end of the couch, take his other leg and position his ankle on your hip. Use your fingers to lock in away from the pubis as you guide the subject into abduction of the hip. This is a great position for treating the adductor magnus, as the subject can move into hip flexion.

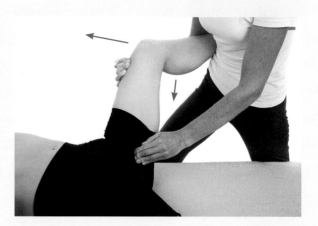

- This can be a ticklish and sensitive area to treat. Ensure that you work within a comfortable ROM.

- If the adductors are particularly tight, shorten, by adducting, prior to locking in.

- Try hooking the opposite leg over the other side of the couch to help maintain the pelvis in neutral.

STR to the adductors in standing:

1) Ensure that the subject is standing with a stable base, feet slightly further than shoulder-width apart. Crouch lateral to his leg and use fingers to lock in and down, away from the pubis into the fibres of the adductor longus. Ask him to flex his opposite knee to initiate a stretch in the muscle.

- This is a very powerful dynamic release and a useful technique to perform at sporting events.

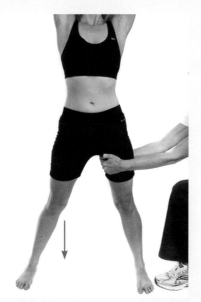
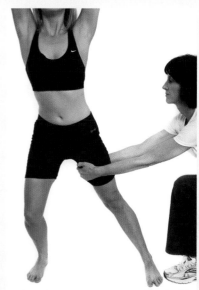

STR to the hamstrings and adductor magnus in standing:

1) Ensure that the subject is standing with a stable base; position one foot facing forwards and the other at 45 degrees. Crouch lateral to his leg, that is at 45 degrees, and use fingers to lock in and down, away from the ischium, into the fibres

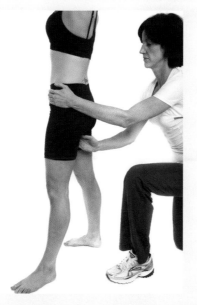
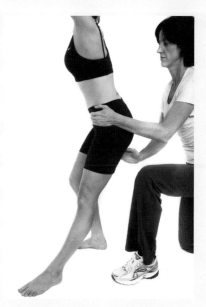

of the hamstrings or adductor magnus. Ask him to flex his opposite knee to initiate a stretch in the muscle; alter the position of the foot to affect the stretch of the muscle that is being addressed.

The Knee

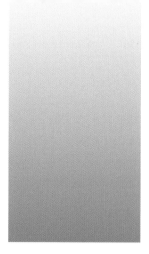

7

As part of the lower limb, the knee has many muscles common to the hip and the ankle and must be examined in a clinical setting as part of that chain. Restriction of a common muscle may have a completely different effect on the knee when compared to either the hip or the ankle.

The knee joint is the tibiofemoral joint, but in the context of this book we will consider the knee joint complex (KJC), which encompasses the following joints:

- tibiofemoral joint
- patellofemoral joint
- proximal tibiofibular joint

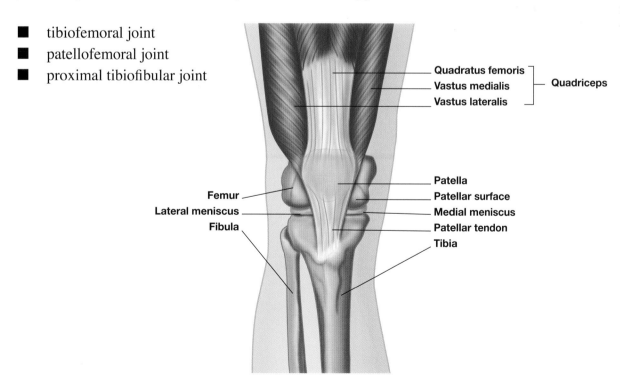

Figure 7.1: Knee joint complex (KJC).

The KJC is one of the most commonly injured joints in sport and everyday slips and falls, partly because of its essential role in ambulation and its reduced stability when compared to the hip. The KJC is the largest joint in the body, and level walking produces an average peak force of three times body weight through each joint.

Movement of the KJC

Tibiofemoral Joint

Often the tibiofemoral joint is seen as a simple hinge joint that is only capable of flexion and extension. The reality is that the arthrokinematics and the osteokinematics are far from being characteristic of a simple hinge joint, as a result of differences between the shapes of the medial and lateral femoral condyles, the menisci, Q angles and muscle structure.

A basic evaluation of the tibiofemoral joint gives the typical ROM measured in an open-chain situation by looking at movement of the tibia on the femur.

Extension	0 to -2 (hyperextension) degrees	Flexion	140 degrees

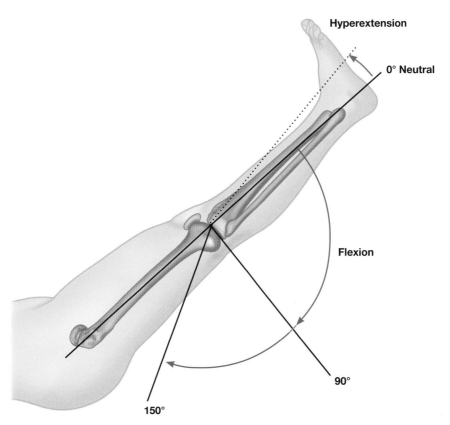

Figure 7.2: Range of motion of the knee.

In everyday life, knee movement is often seen as a closed-chain movement with the foot fixed and the femur moving relative to the tibia, as in sitting down on a chair or squatting. Movement of the knee in these situations is highly associated with movement at the ankle and hip.

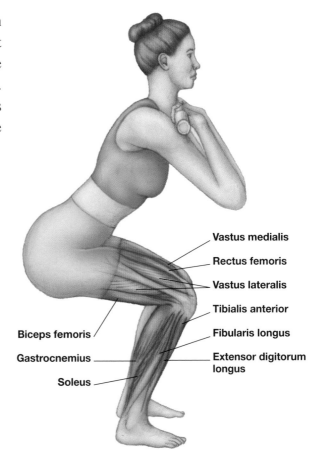

Vastus medialis
Rectus femoris
Vastus lateralis
Tibialis anterior
Fibularis longus
Extensor digitorum longus
Biceps femoris
Gastrocnemius
Soleus

Figure 7.3: Closed-chain knee motion.

Three-dimensional evaluations of the tibia and the femur demonstrate that flexion starts with lateral rotation of the femur, with concomitant femoral rolling and translation (gliding) along all axes. The tibiofemoral joint therefore exhibits six degrees of freedom.

	Femoral motion		Tibial motion	
	Rolling	Rotation	Rolling	Rotation
Flexion	Backward	Lateral	Forward	Medial
Extension	Forward	Medial	Backward	Lateral

Table 7.1: Tibiofemoral motion.

The amount of anterior-posterior femoral translation is subject to debate, with values varying from very little up to 2 cm. This will vary between individuals, but the key point to note is that this movement is likely to be necessary no matter how little or how much it occurs. The anterior-posterior translation is limited by cruciate ligaments, whereas the medial and lateral translation is limited by articular shape, menisci, ligaments and other soft tissue.

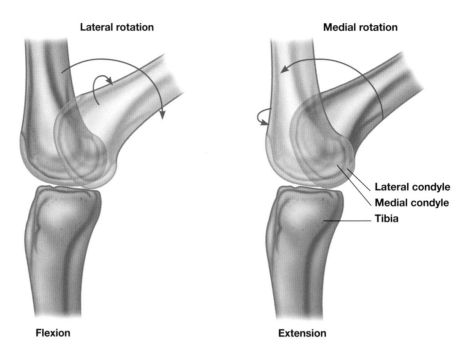

Figure 7.4: Flexion of the femur on the tibia – roll with anterior translation.

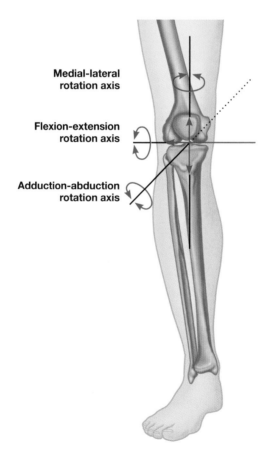

Figure 7.5: Rotation and translation of the knee.

The Screw-Home Mechanism

To maintain stability when walking and to remove quadriceps activity when standing erect, the knee has a unique movement known as the 'screw-home mechanism'. In passive or active knee extension, rotation occurs between the tibia and the femur from full extension to 20 degrees of flexion. The tibia internally rotates with the swing phase and externally rotates with the stance phase; this motion is combined with tightening of the cruciate ligaments.

With the knee flexed, the amount of lateral and medial rotation is difficult to measure: estimates vary between 12 and 80 degrees, and there is virtually no rotation with a fully extended knee. During gait, the estimated rotation is between 8 and 15 degrees. Medial rotation occurs in the stance phase; lateral rotation, in the swing phase.

Patellofemoral Joint

The patellofemoral joint comprises the articulation between the patella and the femur. The shape of the underside of the patella is formed from two facets and a central ridge, which slides between the sulcus formed from the femoral condyles. Its movement is critical for tibiofemoral motion, although it has only two key movements: translation and rotation.

The patella has distal-proximal and lateral-medial translation. It moves distally with knee flexion, combined with limited medial translation at the onset of flexion. Some estimates put distal glide at 7 cm.

Rotation of the patella is not well understood, but the general consensus is that it is capable of rotation around both medial-lateral and anterior-posterior axes.

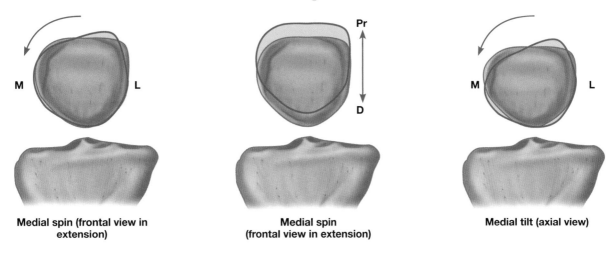

Medial spin (frontal view in extension)	**Medial spin (frontal view in extension)**	**Medial tilt (axial view)**

Figure 7.6: Patella motion.

Proximal Tibiofibular Joint

Flexion and extension of the knee occur with tibial rotation. To allow internal and external rotation of the tibia, motion takes place between the tibia and the fibula: anterior-posterior translation, superior-inferior translation and rotation. These movements are coupled and depend on the position of the knee and ankle joints. There is limited research to quantify movement, and the clinician should assume that if movement here is affected, the overall KJC motion will be too.

Knee Joint Muscles

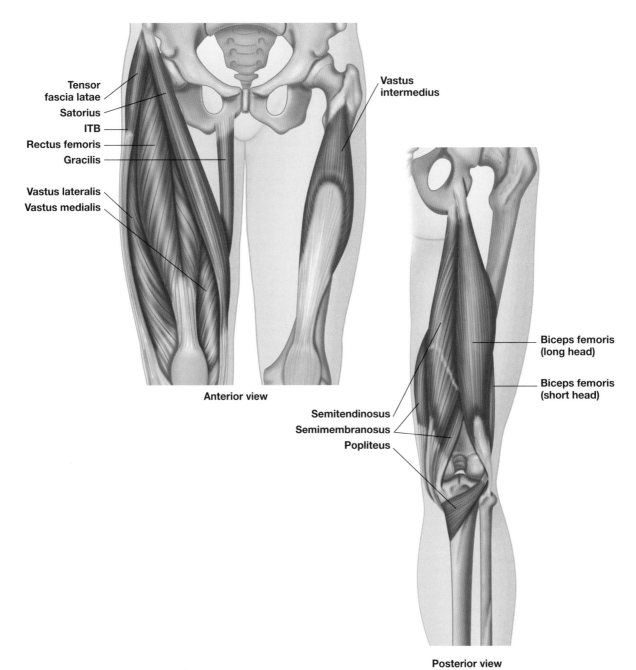

Figure 7.7: Knee joint muscles.

Muscle	Movement of the knee			
	Internal (medial) rotation	External (lateral) rotation	Flexion	Extension
Quadriceps				
Rectus femoris				
Vastus lateralis				
Vastus intermedius				
Vastus medialis				
Hamstrings				
Semimembranosus	Knee, Tibia			
Semitendinosus	Knee, Tibia			
Biceps femoris		Knee, Fibula/Tibia		
Other				
Popliteus	Tibia			
Sartorius				
Gracilis				
Tensor fasciae latae				

Key	Primary role	Secondary role	Possible role

Table 7.2: Muscle movement at the knee joint.

Muscle	Effect of restriction
Quadriceps: Rectus femoris	A common problem causes restriction of the combined movement of the knee (flexion) and hip (extension). Potential increase in pelvic tilt and compensatory increased lumbar extension. Influences gait and stride length. Increased pressure of patella on the femoral condyles with knee flexion and altered patella motion.
Quadriceps: Vastus lateralis Vastus intermedius Vastus medialis	Uncommon, but each would increase pressure on patella with knee flexion, alter patellofemoral motion and limit knee flexion independent of hip position.
Hamstrings: Biceps femoris Semitendinosus Semimembranosus	All of the individual muscles making up the hamstrings are two-joint muscles crossing the hip and knee. Any restriction will limit knee extension, more so with a flexed hip. Individual tightness in semimembranosus and semitendinosus will alter rotation of knee. The biceps femoris has a direct connection to the fibula head and tightness would influence tibiofibular motion. The insertion of the hamstrings to the ischial tuberosity means that tightness may restrict lumbopelvic motion, with consequences on the sacroiliac joint. All of this will affect ambulation, and performance in most sports.
Popliteus	Potentially limits lateral rotation of the tibia or increases medial rotation of the lower leg on the thigh, with consequences on the screw-home mechanism and overall knee efficiency.
Gracilis	Tightness may cause slight flexion contracture and medial rotation of the knee. Little research about effects of isolated restriction of gracilis on the knee, but likely to occur in conjunction with other muscles.
Sartorius	Little research about effects of on isolated basis.
Tensor fasciae latae/iliotibial band (ITB)	Affects the combined hip and knee motion, producing lateral and anterior knee pain via its connection through the ITB and retinaculum. Can cause difficulty with knee extension and lateral patella tracking issues.

Table 7.3: Effects of muscle restrictions on knee movement.

Effects of Knee Muscle Restrictions in Sport and Everyday Life

Running

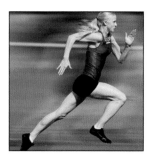

Assuming that the feet and ankles are not the cause of any problems, tightness of the hamstrings could reduce the stride length by limiting knee extension or could increase the force required (by the quadriceps) to achieve knee extension. Individual tightness in the semimembranosus or semitendinosus will affect the rotation of the lower limb on the femur necessary for stability and foot positioning with running gait. All of these effects reduce the efficiency of running, whether sprinting or long distance, and are implicated in many injury scenarios. One study found that "increased hamstring extensibility may improve knee extensor efficiency at heelstrike by enabling greater tibial external rotation and protect the ACL [anterior cruciate ligament] at peak knee flexion by decreasing the tibial internal rotation magnitude".

Rowing

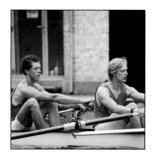

A common problem for rowers is chondromalacia patellae, or wearing of the underside of the patella cartilage. Rowing requires complete knee flexion, and a powerful extension involving the quadriceps. One study calculated that knee joint contact force during extension was 4100 N, or equivalent to over six times body weight. Any restriction in the quadriceps will limit the ability of the rower to fully flex the knee and will increase the joint contact force pushing the patella down onto the femoral condyles, thus leading to or aggravating chondromalacia patellae.

Walking

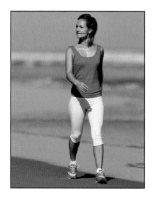

Everyday walking is something taken for granted until there is a problem. Restrictions of quadriceps and hamstrings can affect how we walk and how easy it is for us to perform this activity. Restrictions in the quadriceps will reduce the ability to flex the knee, which may make stepping over raised objects difficult and require more hip flexion. Restricted hamstrings will shorten stride and make fast walking difficult and energy intensive. For older people, who have less muscle strength, this can prove debilitating.

Soft Tissue Release to the Knee

Make a note of the subject's standing position. Check through his passive and active ROM: flexion, extension and rotation. Check the semi-squat in standing and ensure that his knee is flexing over the second toe.

STR to the quadriceps (and TFL) in seated:

1) Position the subject seated at the end of the couch. Use a broad lock, such as a soft fist, to apply a pressure into the quadriceps; ask the subject to flex his knee under the couch. If preferred, start with the leg in an extended position for a fuller ROM.

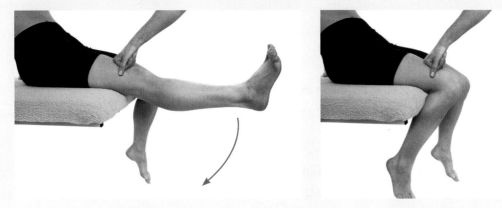

- Ensure that the posterior knee is not impinged on the edge of the couch.

2) Use fingers to lock between the borders of the rectus femoris and the vastus lateralis and between the rectus femoris and the vastus medialis. To reach the borders of the vastus intermedius, gently move the rectus femoris to the side. Ask the subject to flex his knee under the couch.

3) To achieve a greater stretch on the rectus femoris, ask the subject to lie back on the couch, with one knee still over the end; put his other leg up with the foot resting on the couch to protect his back from over lordosis. Lock into the rectus femoris and ask him to flex his knee.

4) Use a thumb reinforced with fingers to gently lock in across the tendon of the origin of the rectus femoris; ask him to flex his knee.

5) Engage the TFL with a soft fist and a CTM lock and ask the subject to flex his knee under the couch.

STR to the quadriceps in supine:

1) Position the subject in supine with the hip slightly flexed and a bolster under the knee. Holding the ankle, extend the knee and lock into the quadriceps, away from the patella; flex the knee.

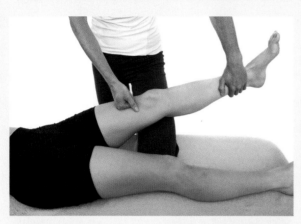 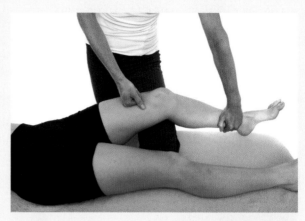

2) This can be done actively by locking in the extended position and asking the subject to flex his knee. Lock away from the patella; address the borders of the vastus muscles.

3) Gently grasp the 'tear drop' vastus medialis and move into a CTM lock, to clear its borders with the rectus femoris and the sartorius. Work with care on the medial border, as it is sensitive.

- Skilled use of the lock will provide a significant release with even a minimal flexion of the knee.

STR to the anterior knee in supine:

1) Use fingers to perform a CTM lock into the medial and lateral patellar retinaculums: lock close to the patella and draw the tissue laterally a few centimetres, maintaining the same pressure. Ask the subject to flex his knee.

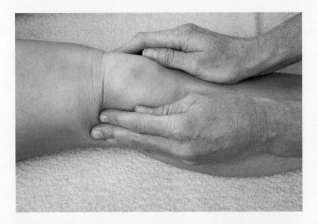 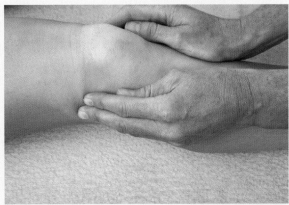

2) Use a knuckle to apply a CTM lock across the patellar tendon: lock in and move the knuckle laterally about a centimetre. Ask the subject to flex his knee.

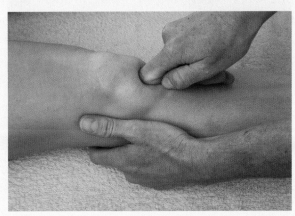

STR to the quadriceps in side lying – freeing up the ITB:

1) Use a soft fist to lock in distally to the vastus lateralis and ask the subject to flex his knee, progressing up the entire muscle.

2) Apply CTM locks, using a thumb reinforced with the other one, and slowly lock into the border between the vastus lateralis and the anterior surface of the ITB; ask the subject to flex his knee. Apply locks in the same way posterior to the ITB; curl up under the ITB to reach the vastus lateralis and ask the subject to flex his knee.

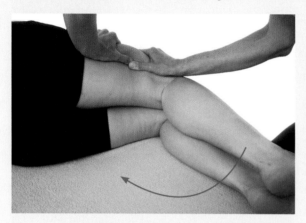 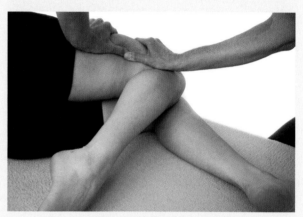

- This is ideal for separating the borders of the vastus lateralis and ITB and will assist in the relief of ITB friction syndrome (see also STR to lateral knee).

- Release of tightness and restriction, particularly of the lateral compartment, aids faulty patellar tracking conditions.

STR to the knee in weight bearing:

1) With the subject standing, use fingers to lock into the medial and lateral patellar retinaculums; ask him to flex a few degrees into a semi-squat.

- This is a very useful tool to assist with the re-education of patellar tracking following any issues with this function.

2) Use a thumb reinforced to apply a lock into the quadriceps, up from the patella; ask the subject to flex into a semi-squat.

3) With the subject standing with his knees in a semi-squat, grasp the tendon of the biceps femoris and ask him to stand up; guide him into medial rotation during extension as necessary. Grasp the pes anserinus and ask him to stand up, guiding him into lateral rotation of the knee as necessary.

STR to the hamstrings in prone:

1) Flex the knee and grasp the ankle; lock into the hamstrings with the heel of a hand or with a soft fist and extend the knee.

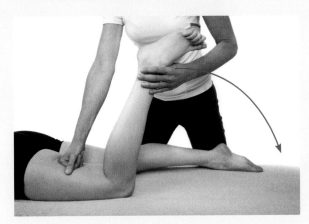 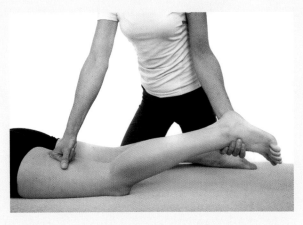

2) This can be done efficiently with active STR. Lock into the belly of the muscle; use fingers to lock into the borders of the biceps femoris, semitendinosus and semimembranosus; ask the subject to extend his knee. Use a knuckle or reinforced thumb for the belly of the muscles.

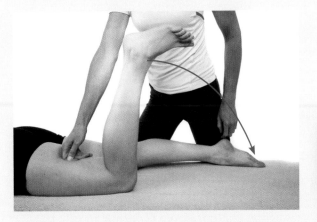 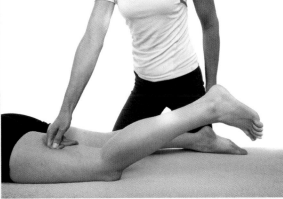

STR to the posterior knee (hamstrings and pes anserinus) in prone:

1) With the knee flexed, grasp the tendon of the biceps femoris and slowly extend the knee; add in a medial rotation of the knee for an extra stretch. Ensure that a lock is performed close to the fibula attachment.

2) With the knee flexed, lock into the semimembranosus located between the tendons of the semitendinosus and the gracilis, and extend the knee. Add in medial rotation of the knee during extension for extra movement.

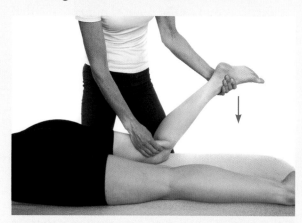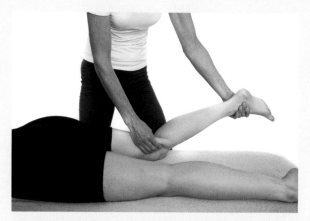

3) With the knee flexed, use fingers to perform a CTM lock on the semitendinosus; just medial to this tendon is the gracilis, and medial again, the sartorius. After each lock, extend the knee. These three muscles merge into the pes anserinus, which can be easily grasped as the subject extends his knee.

- Active STR will help to locate and differentiate these tendons; try supporting the leg during these active movements if the subject finds it too uncomfortable.

STR to the posterior knee (gastrocnemius, popliteus and plantaris) in prone:

1) Grasp the ankle and semi-flex the knee; gently grasp the gastrocnemius origin, between the hamstring tendons, and slowly extend the knee. Do one at a time.

2) Ensure that the gastrocnemius and soleus have been released. With the knee flexed, use fingers to slowly acquire a lock deep to the medial head of the gastrocnemius and into the popliteus; extend the knee.

3) Grasp the ankle and semi-flex the knee. Use fingers to lock into the plantaris, in between the heads of the gastrocnemius; extend the knee.

- The posterior knee can be extremely sensitive, especially around the medial head of the gastrocnemius, so apply locks particularly slowly.

STR to the hamstrings in side lying:

1) Use fingers to lock into the hamstrings while securing the thigh on the other side to ensure that no hip movement takes place; ask the subject to extend his knee.

- This is a useful position for tighter than average hamstrings.

STR to the knee in side lying:

1) Lateral knee: position the subject in side lying with the upper knee semi-flexed on a bolster and the underneath hip extended but knee still semi-flexed. Grasp the tendon of the biceps femoris and ask the subject to extend his knee; use a CTM lock to move across the head of the fibula and ask him to minimally extend his knee. With a reinforced thumb, lock into the lateral head of the subject's gastrocnemius and ask him to extend his knee. Grasp either side of the ITB and ask him to flex his knee.

2) Medial knee: in the same position as above, palpate the underneath knee on the medial side. Gently grasp the pes anserinus tendon and ask the subject to extend his knee. Use a CTM lock across the proximal medial shaft of the tibia and ask him to minimally extend his knee. Lock in medially to the vastus medialis into the sartorius and between the other medial tendons prior to where they merge into the pes anserinus; ask him to extend his knee.

STR to the posterior knee in supine:

1) Use fingers to hook up under the medial and lateral tendons of the posterior knee as the knee is gently flexed. Either passively let the knee drop into extension or ask the subject to slowly extend by pushing down into the fingers.

- Careful application of the lock will allow you to distinguish and separate the tendons.

STR to the hamstrings in supine:

1) Position the subject with his hip flexed and thigh vertical, and his lower leg resting on your shoulder. Apply a lock and ask him to slowly extend his knee within a comfortable range. A variety of locks could be used here depending on how loose the hamstring is and how close the lock is to the tendon attachments.

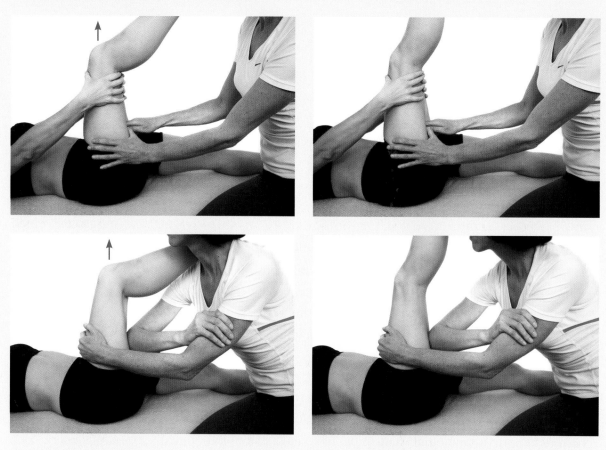

- This is a superb position for hamstring release but ensure that a good position has been established prior to any movement. Consider the flexibility of the hamstrings: if the range is significantly less than 90 degrees, then side lying STR may be a more effective option to allow for full knee extension.

- Support the thigh with the opposite hand to the one applying the lock, or ask the subject to hold his leg during knee extension.

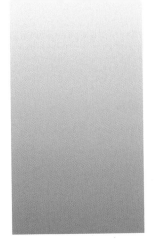

The Ankle and Foot

8

As part of the lower limb, the ankle has some muscles common to the knee and must be examined in a clinical setting as part of the lower limb chain from the hip to the knee to the ankle.

The ankle joint complex includes the:

■ distal (inferior) tibiofibular joint
■ ankle (talocrural) joint
■ subtalar (talocalcaneal) joint

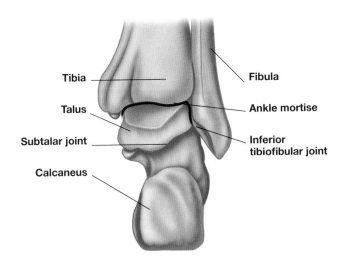

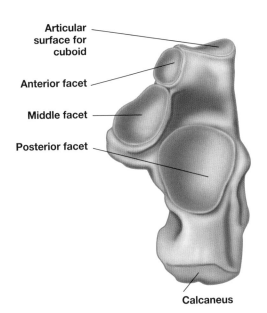

Figure 8.1: The ankle joint complex (posterior view).

A detailed examination of the motion at each joint in the ankle joint complex is beyond the scope and requirements of this book. This section will outline the gross, or osteokinematic, motion made possible by muscles acting on the ankle joint complex that link the foot to the lower limb and specific essential motion created or controlled by extrinsic and intrinsic foot muscles.

The foot is intricately linked to the ankle, with many of the muscles acting on the ankle also controlling movement of the foot. It is therefore sensible to consider both structures together in this section.

The foot comprises the following joints:

- transverse tarsal (Chopart's)
- tarsometatarsal
- metatarsophalangeal (MTP)
- interphalangeal (IP)

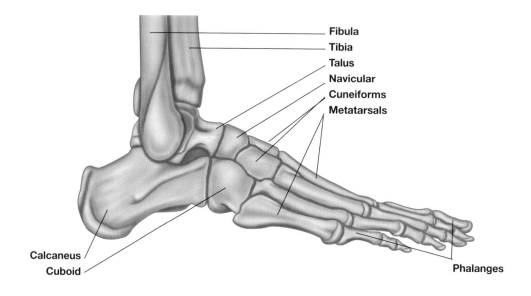

Figure 8.2: The foot.

Motion of the Ankle Joint Complex

Descriptions of ankle joint motion in the literature are often inconsistent and will therefore be kept simple in this text. Ankle joint movement is represented by motion of the foot with respect to the lower limb and falls into three distinct categories, acting in the planes around three axes.

Motion	Cardinal plane	Axis
Abduction/adduction	Transverse	Longitudinal axis through the leg
Eversion/inversion	Frontal	Long axis of the foot through the second metatarsal
Dorsiflexion/plantar flexion	Sagittal	Medial-lateral axis passing approximately through the malleoli

Table 8.1: Motion at the ankle joint complex.

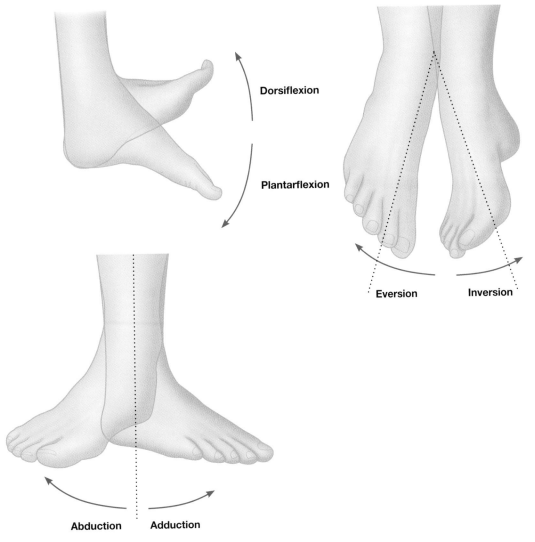

Figure 8.3: Ankle joint range of motion.

Foot and ankle joint motion is complex because, in reality, all three of the categorised motions occur around axes that are oblique to the cardinal planes (see Table 8.1); this motion is referred to as 'tri-planar'. In an open-chain examination (foot free-moving), it is appropriate to use the individual motions in simple clinical tests; however, in closed-chain motion (e.g. walking), it is often more appropriate to examine the motion that occurs as a result of the most common combined movements. These are known as supination and pronation.

Supination	Pronation
Dorsiflexion	Plantar flexion
Eversion	Inversion
Abduction	Adduction

Table 8.2: Supination and pronation

Key Movement at Individual Joints

Joints of the Ankle

Distal tibiofibular joint movement is limited. Whilst there is some rotation of the fibula around a longitudinal axis, with slight proximal-distal and medial-lateral shift, it is all restricted because of the inherent stability required.

The ankle, or talocrural, joint is essentially a hinge joint, with an axis of rotation passing approximately through the malleoli. However, detailed examination shows that this axis of rotation varies according to the amount of plantar flexion and dorsiflexion and is linked to translation of the tibia on the talus.

The subtalar joint, with its three facets on the calcaneus and three domes on the upper surface of the talus, provides a complex pattern of movements that are beyond the scope of this (and many) texts. However, this joint's main role is to enable the ankle to help the foot adapt to uneven terrains by allowing rotation around multiple axes.

Clinically, it has been shown that mobilisation techniques that utilise these natural motions have better outcomes than those methods that do not use them. Muscle restrictions will alter the motion available and change stresses on the bones.

Joints of the Foot

The transverse tarsal joints comprise the talonavicular and calcaneocuboid joints and make up the midfoot. Their combined function is to amplify the movement at the ankle joint and rear foot, contributing to eversion and inversion.

Tarsometatarsal and intermetatarsal joints have limited mobility by way of their need to provide stability during ambulation.

The metatarsophalangeal joints move primarily in the sagittal plane, providing mainly flexion and extension but some rotation and translation. The big toe is required to hyperextend by between 40 and 90 degrees when walking; any reduction in this can lead to structural changes as a result of altered gait and stresses on underlying soft tissue.

Although not a muscle, the foot depends on the plantar fascia working with the big toe to maintain structural integrity through the Windlass mechanism. Failure of this mechanism can lead to many foot problems and issues with intrinsic foot muscles as well as the plantar fascia.

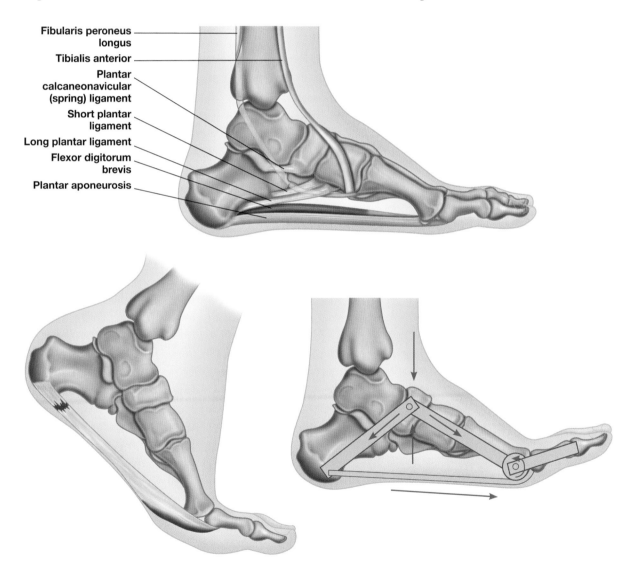

Figure 8.4: Windlass mechanism and the plantar fascia.

Muscles of the Ankle and Foot

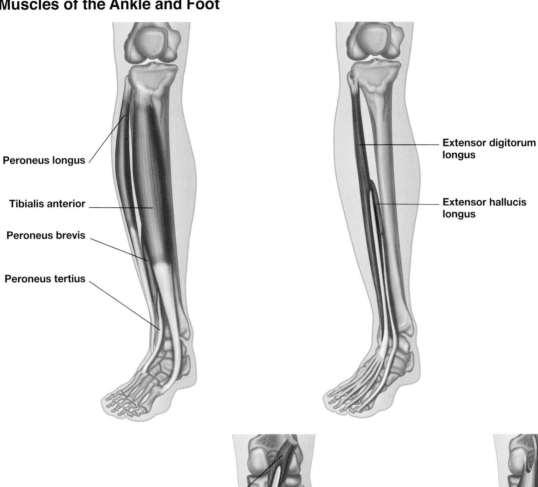

Peroneus longus

Tibialis anterior

Peroneus brevis

Peroneus tertius

Extensor digitorum longus

Extensor hallucis longus

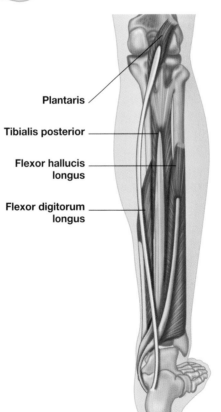

Plantaris

Tibialis posterior

Flexor hallucis longus

Flexor digitorum longus

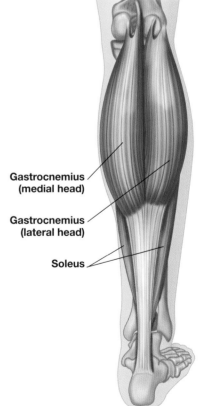

Gastrocnemius (medial head)

Gastrocnemius (lateral head)

Soleus

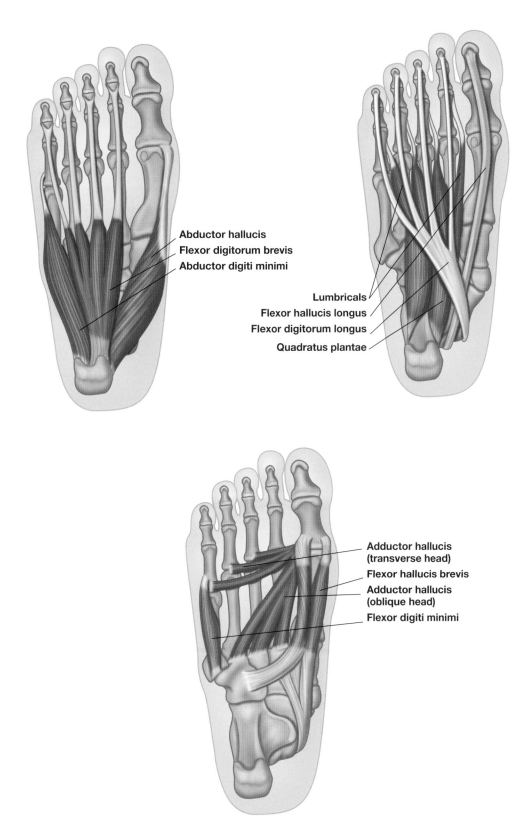

Figure 8.5: Muscles associated with movement of the ankle and foot.

Muscle	Movement of the foot through the ankle					
	Plantar flexion	Dorsiflexion	Abduction	Adduction	Eversion	Inversion
Gastrocnemius	Primary					Secondary
Soleus	Primary					Secondary (Subtalar joint)
Tibialis posterior	Primary					Primary (Subtalar joint)
Flexor digitorum longus	Secondary					Primary (Subtalar joint)
Flexor hallucis longus	Secondary			Secondary		Secondary
Peroneus longus	Secondary		Secondary		Primary	
Plantaris	Primary					Secondary (Subtalar joint)
Peroneus brevis	Secondary				Primary	
Tibialis anterior		Primary				Possible
Extensor hallucis longus		Primary		Secondary		Possible
Extensor digitorum longus		Primary			Possible	
Peroneus tertius		Primary				

Muscle	Movement of the toes			
	Flexion	Extension	Abduction	Adduction
Extensor digitorum brevis (first to fourth toes)		Primary		
Flexor digitorum longus (second to fifth toes)	Primary			
Flexor hallucis longus (big toe)	Primary			
Abductor digiti minimi (fifth toe)			Primary	
Quadratus plantaris (second to fifth toes)	Primary			
Lumbricals (second to fifth toes)	Primary			

Key	Primary role	Secondary role	Possible role

Table 8.3: Muscle movement at the ankle and foot.

Muscle	Effect of restriction/tightness
Gastrocnemius	Because it is a two-joint muscle, the effect will depend on the relative positions of the knee and ankle. ROM is increased with a flexed knee. When standing, tightness may prevent heel contact and contribute to toe walking. It will also impact on gait during stance and swing phases.
Achilles tendon	The Achilles tendon is mentioned as it is the largest tendon in the body and an important soft tissue structure for locomotion. Any tightness here will reduce transmission of force from the gastrocnemius and make it prone to injury through reduction in tensile strength. It may also pull on the calcaneus, creating a hindfoot inversion (ankle varus).
Soleus	Prevents normal motion of the tibia over the foot in gait and can lead to development of genu recurvatum or postural lean-back when standing.
Tibialis posterior	Results in foot inversion and adduction and potential equinovarus deformity.
Plantaris	No known specific effect, although it may be affected by tightness of the tibialis posterior and add to plantar flexion deformity.
Peroneus longus	May affect inversion at the subtalar joint and create a plantar flexed first ray with potential for observed supination in stance.
Peroneus brevis	Individually, little potential effect but could contribute to valgus of hindfoot.
Tibialis anterior	Development of pes cavus foot shape (high arch), due to pull of the muscle on the medial longitudinal arch.
Extensor hallucis longus	Creates extension at the MTP joint of the big toe, causing the IP joint to flex, resulting in claw toe and abnormal stress on the MTP when walking.
Extensor digitorum longus	Creates extension at the MTP and flexion at the IP joints, with the development of claw toes, leading to pain and limitation of normal function.
Peroneus tertius	Unlikely to have a significant effect.
Flexor digitorum longus (second to fifth toes)	Reduced extension of the toes and a factor in the development of claw toe deformity.
Flexor hallucis longus (big toe)	Reduces extension of the big toe, particularly when the ankle is in dorsiflexion. Can contribute to claw toe in the big toe.
Abductor digiti minimi (fifth toe) Quadratus plantaris (second to fifth toes) Lumbricals (second to fifth toes) Extensor digitorum brevis (first to fourth toes)	There are few (if any) studies on the impact of tightness of the intrinsic muscles of the foot. However, their role in stabilising the foot during gait means that any localised tightness could affect the function of the foot.

Table 8.4: Effects of muscle restrictions on ankle and foot movement.

Effects of Ankle Muscle Restrictions in Sport and Everyday Life

Rugby

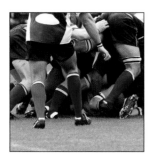

Studies of professional rugby players have found correlations between stress fractures of the metatarsals and Achilles tendon contracture and limited dorsiflexion of the ankle, subtalar joint or both. There are also studies linking midfoot and/or forefoot overuse symptoms to increased tightness in the gastrocnemius and soleus.

Volleyball

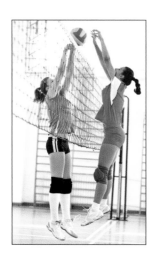

One study has found that players with patellar tendinopathy had significantly lower ankle dorsiflexion range than players with normal tendons, and that a range of ankle dorsiflexion of less than 45 degrees appeared to increase the risk of patellar tendinopathy by a factor of 1.8–2.8, compared to normal tendons.

In volleyball an inversion sprain is also common, in which injury often occurs to the peroneus longus muscle. If allowed to develop scar tissue, this muscle will lose its normal function, which is key to ankle stability on landing. Any instability developed is then more likely to lead to repeat injuries.

Common Foot Problems

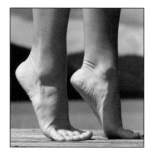

Tightness in many of the ankle and intrinsic foot muscles will cause changes in the shape of the foot – including claw toes, cavus foot and supination – all of which affect its ability to function normally. This can lead to increased pressure on the metatarsal heads, and the development of hard skin and pain from pressure on shoes.

Soft Tissue Release to the Ankle

Make a note of the subject's standing position. Check through his active and passive ROM.

STR to the superficial posterior compartment (gastrocnemius, soleus, and plantaris) in prone:

1) Position the subject in prone with his ankles off the end of the couch. Use fingers to lock into the gastrocnemius, between the bellies; gently flex his ankle with your own knee.

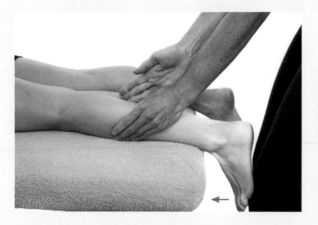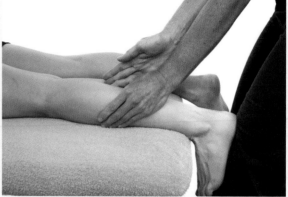

Use fingers to lock in, between the bellies, and ask him to flex his ankle.

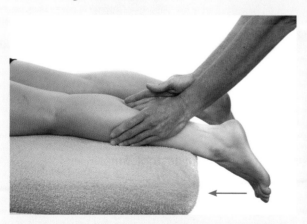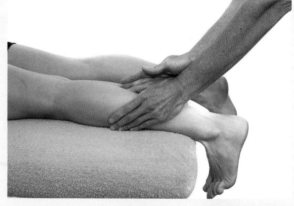

Lock into the belly of the muscle, curl under the lateral and medial borders of the muscle, clearing any restriction with the soleus; ask him to flex his ankle. Gently pick up the paratenon of the Achilles; ask him to flex his ankle.

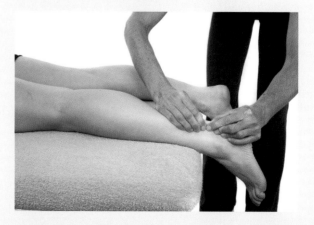

2) With his knee flexed to 90 degrees, cup his heel with one hand. Use fingers to lock into the soleus, deep to the gastrocnemius; gently flex his ankle. Locate the medial and lateral portions of the soleus that emerge from the gastrocnemius and flex the ankle.

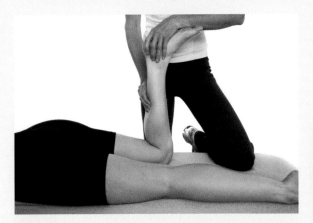 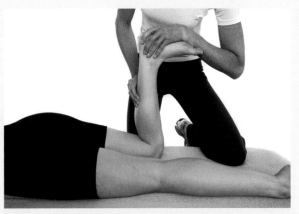

3) Position the subject in prone with his knee flexed and one knee under your anterior lower leg. Lock in and ask him to flex his ankle. Grasp the distal portion of the soleus; use fingers to pick up the paratenon. Ask him to flex his ankle.

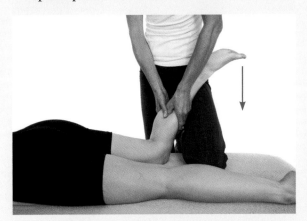 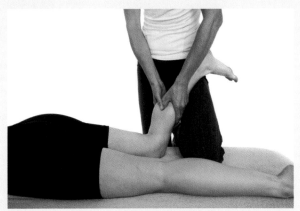

- Thorough release of these muscles and fascia will contribute to the healing of Achilles tendinopathies; clearing restriction enables effective strengthening.

STR around the medial and lateral malleoli in prone:

1) Use a knuckle to apply a CTM lock away from the lateral malleolus; ask the subject to dorsiflex his ankle.

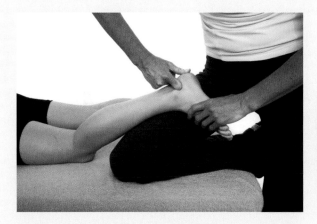 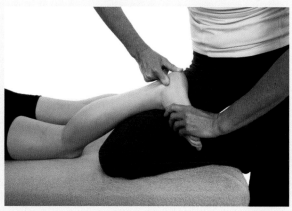

2) Use a knuckle to apply a CTM lock away from the medial malleolus; ask the subject to dorsiflex his ankle.

- Try two or three locks, each in a different direction, away from each malleolus.

STR to the superficial posterior compartment in side lying:

1) Use fingers to drop in between the gastrocnemius and soleus; ask him to dorsiflex his ankle. This can be done on the lateral and medial borders.

STR to the superficial compartment in weight bearing:

1) With the subject standing with one leg forward and leaning on a solid surface, lock into the closest calf muscle. Ask him to lunge forwards for a gastrocnemius stretch and ask him to flex both knees for a soleus stretch.

2) With the subject standing, try locking in with the heel plantar flexed; ask him to drop his heel to the ground, with the knee either straight or bent.

STR to the deep posterior compartment (tibialis posterior, flexor digitorum longus and flexor hallucis longus) in prone:

1) Ensure that the superficial compartment is relaxed and warmed up. Position the subject with his knee flexed and one knee under his anterior lower leg. Lock in, deep to the superficial compartment, with a reinforced thumb or a knuckle; ask him to flex his ankle.

2) Position the subject with the knee flexed and his lower leg vertical and supported. Tweeze in with fingers, deep to the superficial compartment; ask him to flex his ankle.

STR to the deep posterior compartment (tibialis posterior, flexor digitorum longus and flexor hallucis longus) in side lying:

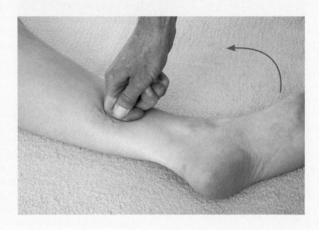

1) Flex the hip and knee of the upper leg (place a support under the knee) to expose the underneath leg. Use knuckles to lock in away from the lower third of the medial tibia and ask him to dorsiflex his ankle.

   • Carefully acquire a lock, since if this area is congested, it will be very sensitive; avoid direct contact with any acute area directly on the periosteum or in the surrounding tissue.

2) Lock in away from the medial malleolus and move posteriorly to address the distal bellies and tendons; dorsiflex the ankle.

STR to the lateral compartment (peroneus longus and peroneus brevis) in supine:

1) Stand on the opposite side of the couch. Start from the head of the fibula and hook fingers into the peroneus longus; ask the subject to dorsiflex or invert his ankle. Address the upper two-thirds of the lateral surface of the fibula for the peroneus longus and the lower third for the peroneus brevis; ask him to dorsiflex his ankle.

2) Curl fingers around the lateral malleolus and ask him to dorsiflex his ankle.

STR to the lateral compartment (peroneus longus and peroneus brevis) in side lying:

1) Use a reinforced thumb to apply a CTM lock away from the head of the fibula; ask him to dorsiflex his ankle. Apply locks across the lateral surface of the fibula; ask him to dorsiflex his ankle.

2) Use fingers to separate the borders between the peroneus longus and the soleus; ask him to dorsiflex his ankle. Use fingers to apply a CTM lock away from the lateral border of the fibula and towards the anterior surface of the fibula, in between the peroneus longus and the extensor digitorum longus; ask him to dorsiflex his ankle.

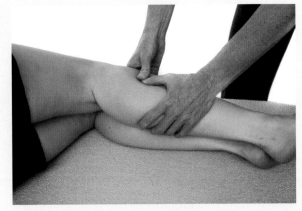

- Pay attention to the area around the head of the fibula for a maximum release.

STR to the anterior compartment (tibialis anterior, extensor digitorum longus, peroneus tertius, when present, and extensor hallucis longus) in supine:

1) Use knuckles to lock into the tibialis anterior; ask the subject to plantar flex his ankle. Dorsiflex the ankle prior to locking for a greater range.

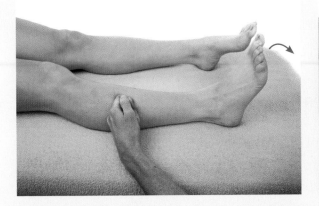 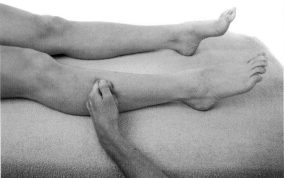

Use fingers to gently grasp the tendon of insertion and plantar flex the ankle.

- A CTM lock is ideal in the muscle of the tibialis anterior, as the myofascia is particularly dense.

- Try a lateral lock by locking in and away from the tibia.

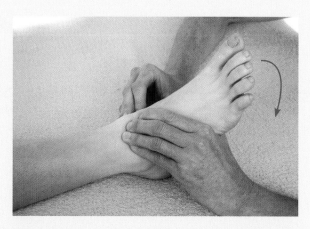

3) From the side of the couch, use fingers or a reinforced thumb to lock into the extensor digitorum longus, in between the tibialis anterior and peroneus longus; ask the subject to plantar flex his foot. Follow the muscle down to the retinaculum and lock into the tendon; ask him to plantar flex his ankle.

4) Use fingers to lock into the tendons on the top of the foot and ask him to plantar flex his ankle. Lock into the hallucis longus, between the extensor digitorum longus and the tibialis anterior; lock into the tendon on the surface of the big toe; plantar flex the ankle.

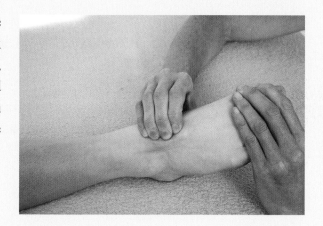

Ankle sprains and strains

Following any type of ankle sprain, all of the lower leg muscle compartments and the foot need to be systematically addressed. Gentle STR can be applied in the sub-acute stage of rehabilitation, avoiding any inflamed areas; early treatment will minimise scarring, thickening and muscle imbalance. In the chronic stage more vigorous STR may be necessary. Ensure that STR is conducted at the muscle borders, across the retinaculum and away from the malleoli. Skilled use of active STR will help restore normal movement and provide appropriate proprioceptive re-education for the subject.

Pay particular attention to the lateral compartment of the peroneus longus and brevis. These muscles act to prevent inversion and therefore protect against ankle inversion sprains.

Soft Tissue Release to the Foot

The layers of different muscles in the foot offer stability for the body and also provide fine movement and plyometric strength for propulsion. Make a note of the subject's natural standing position and presentation of the arches. Check passive and active ROM for inversion and eversion separately and in conjunction with dorsiflexion and plantar flexion of the ankle. Check flexion and extension of the toes.

STR to the foot evertors (peroneus longus and peroneus brevis) in supine:

1) From the same side of the couch, lock into the peroneus brevis in the lower third of the lateral fibula, using a thumb reinforced with the other one; ask the subject to invert his foot.

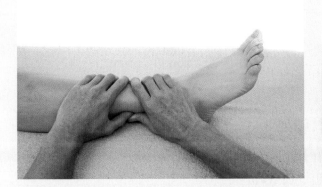 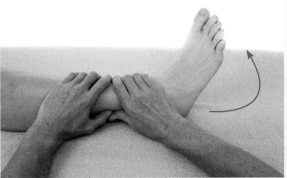

Lock into the belly of the peroneus longus on the upper two-thirds of the lateral surface of the fibula. Use a CTM lock to engage the tendons as they curl behind the lateral malleolus (the longus tendon is slightly posterior to the brevis tendon). Ask the subject to invert his foot. Alternatively, stand on the opposite side of the couch. Hook fingers into the peroneus longus and brevis; ask the subject to invert his foot.

- Perform a CTM lock at the tendon attachment at the base of the first metatarsal and medial cuneiform.

- Consider the tibialis anterior attachment and balance between the peroneus and tibialis anterior muscle in maintenance of the lateral arch; they meet to form a 'stirrup' for the foot.

STR to the foot evertors (peroneus longus and peroneus brevis) in side lying:

1) Use a reinforced thumb to apply a CTM lock away from the head of the fibula; ask him to invert his foot. Address the upper two-thirds of the lateral surface of the fibula for the peroneus longus and the lower third for the peroneus brevis; ask him to invert his foot.

- Apply a CTM lock away from the lateral malleolus.

STR to the foot invertors (tibialis anterior, extensor hallucis longus, tibialis posterior, flexor digitorum longus and flexor hallucis longus) in supine:

1) Use fingers to gently pick up the tendon of insertion of the tibialis anterior; ask him to evert his foot. Lock in away from the middle section of the fibula into the hallucis longus, between the extensor digitorum longus and the tibialis anterior; ask him to evert his foot.

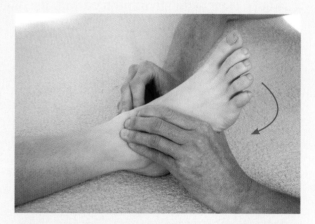

2) Use a reinforced thumb to drop off the medial malleolus into the tendons of the deep posterior compartment: the tibialis posterior is the most anterior and superficial, the flexor digitorum is posterior to it and the flexor hallucis longus is posterior to this, deep to the Achilles. Ask him to evert his foot.

STR to the plantar fascia in supine:

1) Secure the top of the foot with one hand. Use a soft fist to apply pressure with a CTM lock; ask the subject to extend his toes. Start from the toes and perform two or three of these broad surface locks and progress towards the calcaneus.

2) Once the fascia has softened, progress to a deeper, more specific lock using a knuckle.

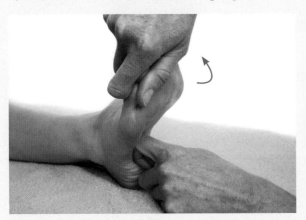 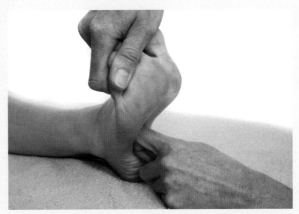

- In the case of plantar fasciitis, a specific lock can be applied very close to the inflamed area on the medial heel, without actually disturbing or irritating it.

- Use a CTM lock to apply locks at different points away from the heel; four layers of fascia emerge from here.

STR to the toe extensors (extensor digitorum longus, extensor digitorum brevis and extensor hallucis longus) in supine:

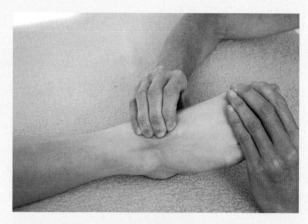

1) Sit at the end of the couch. Use fingers to tweeze in between the tendons of the extensor digitorum longus on the dorsal surface of the four lateral toes; ask the subject to flex his toes. Gently lock into the tendons and ask him to flex his toes.

2) Lock into the belly of the extensor digitorum longus, away from the anterior surface of the fibula; ask him to plantar flex his ankle.

3) Lock into the extensor hallucis longus and ask him to flex his big toe. Try to gently pick up the tendon and ask him to flex his toe.

4) Use fingers to apply pressure into the extensor digitorum brevis, deep to the extensor digitorum longus; passively flex the middle three toes or ask the subject to flex his toes.

- Try to separate any adhesion between the extensor tendons and the retinaculum, by using a superficial CTM lock. Lock in and plantar flex the ankle and flex the toes.

STR to the toe flexors (flexor digitorum longus, flexor digitorum brevis, flexor digitorum accessorius, flexor hallucis longus, flexor hallucis brevis, flexor digiti minimi brevis, lumbricals and interossei) in supine:

1) Use a reinforced thumb, to locate the tendon of the flexor hallucis longus, medial and deep to the Achilles tendon; ask him to extend his big toe. Combine this with dorsiflexion of the ankle as necessary.

   • Flexor hallucis longus plays an important role in maintenance of the medial arch.

2) Use a knuckle to lock into the flexor digitorum brevis; apply locks from the second to fifth toes and work towards the medial tubercle of the heel. Ask him to extend his toes.

3) Use a reinforced thumb to apply a CTM lock at the bases of the proximal phalanges; ask him to extend his toes.

STR to the toe abductors (abductor hallucis, dorsal interossei and abductor minimi) in supine:

1) Grasp the big toe and gently abduct it. Use a knuckle to apply a CTM lock into the abductor hallucis on the medial plantar surface of the foot; gently adduct or extend the big toe.

2) Grasp the little toe and gently abduct it. Use a knuckle to apply a CTM lock into the abductor digiti minimi on the lateral plantar surface of the foot; gently adduct or extend the fifth toe.

   • Try various locks of different depths and location to cover the plantar aspect of the foot. Apply locks close to the toe joints.

STR to toe adductors (adductor hallucis and plantar interossei) in supine:

1) Gently lock in with a thumb at the lateral base of the big toe (proximal phalange); gently abduct the big toe.

2) Use a knuckle to apply a CTM lock into the tendon sheath of the peroneus longus; ask the subject to splay his toes.

- The adductor hallucis is often inhibited and requires strength to maintain the distal transverse arch. Minimal STR to the adductor hallucis will facilitate any strengthening required.

Arches

Maintenance of the arches is dependent on strength and balance of the soft tissues in the foot. Consider the four layers of intrinsic foot muscles and the length and strength of the lower leg muscles. Systematically treating all of the lower leg, the foot muscles and the plantar fascia will enhance functional re-education programmes.

Case Study 1 – Elbow Pain

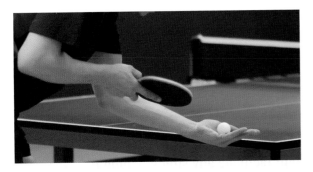

A 59-year-old man in otherwise good health was experiencing bilateral elbow pain. His main hobbies included playing table tennis to a high standard, and helping with woodland development for the National Trust.

Pain around the elbow joints and down into the hands was worse in the morning and after lifting objects while working in woodland development. It was interfering with playing table tennis.

On first impressions, the whole upper body was restricted in movement: the left and right scapulae were protracted, elbow extension was reduced, and supination and pronation of the hand were restricted, especially when performing the dysdiadochokinesia test.

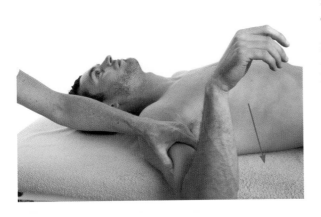

STR

The upper body needed work. The main muscles treated included the biceps, triceps, pectoralis major and minor, anterior deltoid, brachialis, pronator teres and wrist flexors.

The patient was given an STR self-treatment programme for the pronator teres and elbow flexors, and basic stretches for the pectoral muscles.

Outcome

After two sessions the pain had disappeared in both elbows, and playing table tennis was no longer a problem.

Rationale

The position of the arms across the body, and the specific but limited movements in table tennis, coupled with the gripping and lifting in woodland work, had created restrictions in much of the upper limbs and shoulder girdle. This is a good example of when STR should be applied to the kinetic chain involved and not simply to one muscle.

Case Study 2 – Shoulder Girdle

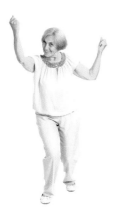

An 89-year-old lady, mentally alert and active and presenting an unremarkable medical history, attended the clinic with a painful and restricted shoulder, diagnosed as a frozen shoulder by her GP. One of her biggest concerns was that she could not brush her hair, and doing the ironing was difficult – she did not trust her husband to do it!

Testing ruled out any major bony or soft tissue impingement and muscle tears. Active lateral abduction of the arm was limited to approximately 90 degrees, with passive being somewhat more.

STR

The main muscles treated were the subscapularis, serratus anterior and trapezius. The pectoralis minor required a little work. She was given some simple stretches for the shoulders.

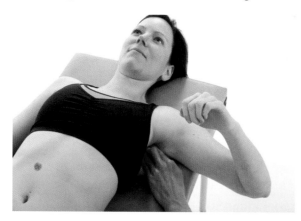
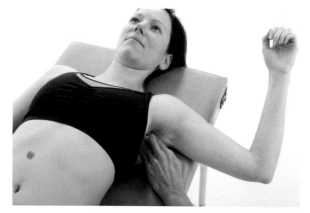

Outcome

After three 30-minute sessions over three weeks she was able to report that she could not only brush her hair and iron but also hang out the washing, which she had not been able to do for a long time. Three months later she returned for a follow-up and was still able to do everything she wanted.

Rationale

Age-related restrictions are very common, as over our lifetimes we develop habits aimed at minimising pain. Often older people are told that age is the problem, whereas in many cases the problem is no different to that affecting younger people – the lack of a full range of motion. This is a great example of how older people can have their life improved by you taking the time to help them understand why the problem has occurred, and starting them on their way back to normal pain-free movement with STR.

Case Study 3 – Hamstrings

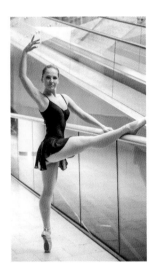

A 17-year-old dancer had injured her hamstrings three weeks earlier when she was moving up from a leg-split position into a front-kick movement. At the time there was bruising at the hamstrings origin. As a young dancer she was concerned about this, since she had an exam in two weeks' time but had been told she could not take it because of the injury.

An assessment indicated a definite hamstring injury at the origin, but the question was, why had it occurred? Moreover, how would it be possible for her to take the exam? Further assessment showed that, while she was flexible, there were areas of restriction in the lumbar muscles, gluteal muscles and mid hamstrings.

STR

The hamstrings underwent precise STR application along their whole length and to each of the component muscles – the semimembranosus, semitendinosus and biceps femoris. In addition, the gluteal muscles, lumbar erector spinae and quadratus lumborum were worked. She was given a seated STR self-treatment programme for the hamstrings, along with stretches for the gluteal muscles.

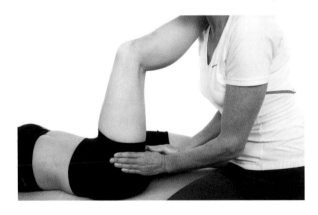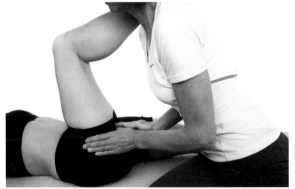

Outcome

She had three sessions within ten days and was seen again four days before her exam, at which time she went through a trial routine without too much difficulty. She later took the exam and passed.

Rationale

Like many dancers she had good overall flexibility, but a distinct area of restriction. In this case, when completing extreme moves quickly, the lumbopelvic rhythm was being disrupted by these restrictions, so that stress was being placed on the weakest areas, namely the upper hamstrings and their origin.

Case Study 4 – Head and Face Pain

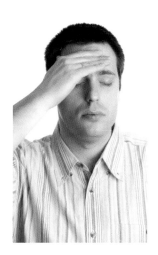

A 44-year-old man presented with head and face pain that had been diagnosed as migraine. An assessment and history analysis suggested that the evidence for diagnosing migraine was weak. The pain became worse during and after activity, and was mainly up one side of the face, around and into the left eye, and onto the forehead. It was particularly pronounced after bench pressing or running.

All of the head, neck and shoulder girdle muscles were assessed, and, although there was some tightness and restriction, it was no more than would be considered normal. However, work on the sternocleidomastoid muscle immediately reproduced the pain that had been diagnosed as migraine.

STR

The generalised muscle tightness in the neck and shoulder was treated, with the focus being on the sternocleidomastoid muscle. An STR self-treatment programme was also given.

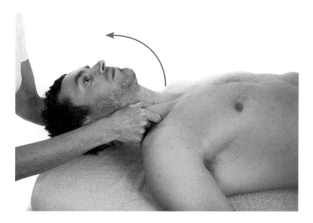
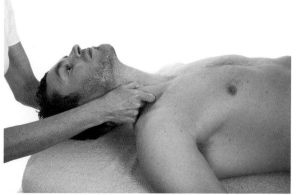

Outcome

Having had the head and face pain for several years, the man was able to train and run without any problems after undergoing three treatments over six weeks, along with an STR self-treatment programme.

Rationale

Referred pain from the muscles of the neck and head has long been known to either imitate a migraine or be a part of the 'triggering' process of the condition. In this case the sternocleidomastoid muscle had shortened, and when stressed was referring pain into the area associated with migraine.

Case Study 5 – Achilles Tendinopathy

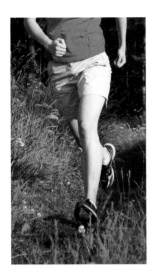

A 42-year-old female club-standard 10k runner covering 35 miles per week had been prescribed enforced rest from running for ten days because of a heavy cold. On resuming training she felt pain in her right Achilles while running and walking, and also first thing in the morning.

An initial investigation indicated no obvious restriction in movement in the lower leg. However, on palpation the lower leg muscles on the right side were sticking at the borders, with obvious congestion at the musculotendinous border between the soleus and the gastrocnemius. The Achilles also presented with minimal swelling and was tender to the touch.

STR

All the lower leg compartments were treated, focusing on the borders in between the musculotendinous junction and the gastrocnemius and soleus muscles.

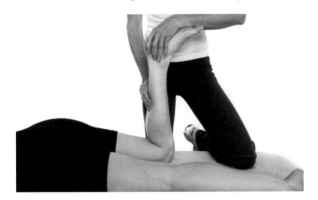
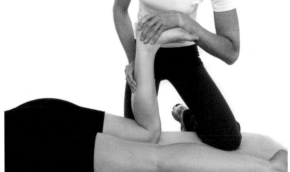

Outcome

The patient felt immediate relief on walking, and was able to run pain-free the following day.

Rationale

The calf complex was not functioning at its optimum because of soft tissue restrictions, and this inefficiency placed undue pressure on the Achilles. The athlete's rest from training and stretching had possibly caused the connective tissues to stiffen a little, consequently affecting the Achilles. Although she was not aware of any problems with her Achilles or calf, it is most likely that the soft tissue restrictions had been present for some time.

She was advised to monitor her calf with STR self-treatment, and to reduce training. It was also recommended that she ice the Achilles until the swelling had dissipated and report back for a fuller assessment if her symptoms reappeared.

Case Study 6 – Groin Pain

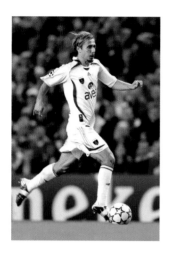

A 35-year-old footballer had been suffering for over six weeks from groin pain following a sliding tackle. He had not been able to resume playing, as he felt a sharp pain in his groin. This would catch him periodically during the day, but was not really a problem unless he tried to run above a jogging speed. He had not had any treatment.

An assessment revealed him to be generally very stiff, particularly in both sets of hamstrings and adductors. The adductors on the affected side were markedly more shortened; stretching them reproduced his pain but to a lesser extent. There was an area of scar tissue and adhesive tissue towards the origin of the adductor longus.

STR

All the adductor muscles were treated with an emphasis on the origins and the area of fibrous tissue, where a gentle CTM lock was applied as he slowly initiated a minimal abduction. The hip musculature in general was addressed, but in particular the hip flexors and the lower back.

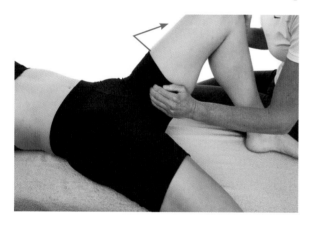
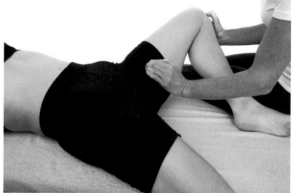

Outcome

The patient felt significant relief on stretching the adductors, and his hips felt 'lighter'. He had two further treatments in which the soft tissue restrictions were released, and the adductor length then matched that of the opposing leg. To help maintain his increased flexibility, he was advised on STR self-treatment and stretching. He was also recommended to consider Pilates to help attain pelvic balance and improve his core strength, which would enable him to continue playing football to an older age.

Rationale

There was an obvious area of fibrous tissue towards the origin of the adductor longus, and an associated tissue restriction in the adductors, which was probably caused by the initial strain and was the primary reason for his pain and reduced movement.

Resources

Books

Adams, M. et al. 2006. *The Biomechanics of Back Pain*. Churchill Livingstone, Edinburgh.

Alter, M. J. 2004. *Science of Flexibility, 3e*. Human Kinetics, Champaign.

Armiger, P. & Martyn, M. A. 2009. *Stretching for Functional Flexibility*. Lippincott, Williams & Wilkins, Baltimore.

Barcsay, J. 1997. *Anatomy for the Artist: A Detailed Portrayal of he Human Body for the Artist*. Little Brown, New York.

Biel, A. 2011. *Trail Guide to the Body: A Hands-On Guide to Locating Muscles, Bones, and more, 4e*. Books of Discovery, Boulder.

Brukner, P. & Khan, K. 2012. *Clinical Sports Medicine, 4e*. McGraw-Hill, New York.

Butler, D. 1991. *Mobilisation of the Nervous System*. Churchill Livingstone, Edinburgh.

Cailliet, R. 1981. *Neck and Arm Pain, Pain Series*. F. A. Davis Co., Philadelphia.

Cailliet, R.1982. *Hand Pain, Pain Series*. F. A. Davis Co., Philadelphia.

Cailliet, R. 1977. *Soft Tissue Pain and Disability, Pain Series*. F. A. Davis Co., Philadelphia.

Cailliet, R. 1983. *Knee Pain, Pain Series*. F. A. Davis Co., Philadelphia.

Cailliet R. 1983. *Foot and Ankle Pain, Pain Series*. F. A. Davis Co., Philadelphia.

Cailliet, R. 1981. *Shoulder Pain, Pain Series*. F. A. Davis Co., Philadelphia.

Cailliet, R. 1980. *Low Back Pain Syndrome, 3e, Pain Series*. F. A. Davis Co., Philadelphia.

Cailliet, R. 2003. *The Illustrated Guide to Functional Anatomy of Musculoskeletal System*. F. A. Davis Co., Philadelphia.

Cantu, R. I. & Grodin, A. J. 1992. *Myofascial Manipulation: Theory and Clinical Application*. Aspen Publishers Inc., Maryland.

Cash, M. 1996. *Sport and Remedial Massage Therapy*. Ebury Press, London.

Chaitow, L. 2006. *Muscle Energy Techniques*. Churchill Livingstone, Edinburgh.

Chaitow, L. 2007. *Positional Release Techniques*. Churchill Livingstone, Edinburgh.

Chaitow, L. 1980. *Soft Tissue Manipulation: A Practitioner's Guide to the Diagnosis and Treatment of Soft Tissue Dysfunction and Reflex Activity*. Healing Arts Press, Vermont.

Cyriax, J. & Cyriax, P. 1996. *Illustrated Manual of Orthopaedic Medicine*. Butterworth-Heinemann, Oxford.

Dryden, T. & Moyer, C. A. 2012. *Massage Therapy, Integrating Research and Practice*. Human Kinetics, Champaign.

Gray, H. 2009. *Gray's Anatomy*. Running Press, Philadelphia.

Juhan, D. 1998. *Job's Body – A Handbook for Bodywork*. Station Hill, Barrytown Limited.

Kendall, F. P. et al. 2010. *Muscles Testing and Function: Testing With Posture and Pain, 5e*. Lippincott, Williams & Wilkins, Baltimore.

Lederman, E. 2005. *The Science and Practice of Manual Therapy*. Churchill Livingstone, Edinburgh

McAtee, B. 2010. *Facilitated Stretching*. Human Kinetics, Champaign.

McGill, S. 2002. *Low Back Disorders*. Human Kinetics, Champaign.

McMinn, R., Hutchings, R.T., Pegington, J. & Abrahams, P.H. 1993. *A Colour Atlas of Human Anatomy*. Wolfe, New York.

McMinn, R. & Hutchings, R. 1982. *Foot and Ankle Anatomy*. Wolfe, New York.

Myers, T.W. 2009. *Anatomy Trains, 2e*. Churchill Livingstone, Edinburgh.

Noakes, T. 1991. *Lore of Running*. Human Kinetics, Champaign.

Norris, C.M. 1993. *Sports Injuries: Diagnosis and Management*. Butterworth-Heinemann, Oxford.

Oatis, C. 2004. *Kinesiology: The Mechanics and Pathomechanics of Human Movement*. Lippincott, Williams & Wilkins, Baltimore.

Plastanga, N. & Soames, R. 2012. *Anatomy and Human Movement: Structure and Function*. Churchill Livingstone, Edinburgh.

Read, M. & Wade, P. 2009. *Sports Injuries: A Unique Guide to Self-Diagnosis and Rehabilitation, 3e*. Churchill Livingstone, Edinburgh.

Rockwood, C.A. et al. 1998. *The Shoulder, Vol. 1*. W.B. Saunders, New York.

Rolf, I. P. 1992. *Rolfing, Re-establishing the Natural Alignment and Structural Integration of the Human Body for Vitality and Well-Being*. Healing Arts Press, Vermont.

Sahrmann, S. A. 2001. *Diagnosis and Treatment of Movement Impairment Syndromes*. Mosby, New York.

Stone, J. & Stone, R. 2011. *Atlas of Skeletal Muscles, 7e*. McGraw-Hill, New York.

Tortora, G. and Grabowski, S.R. 1999. *Principles of Anatomy and Physiology, 9e*. John Wiley & Sons, Chichester.

Watkins, J. 1998. *Structure and Function of the Musculoskeletal System*. Human Kinetics, Champaign.

Whiting, W.C., Zernicke, R.F. 2008. *Biomechanics of Musculoskeletal Injury*. Human Kinetics, Champaign.

Wilmore, J.H. & Costill, D.L. 2007. *Physiology of Sport and Exercise*. Human Kinetics, Champaign.

Wirhed, R. 2006. *Athletic Ability and the Anatomy of Motion*. Mosby, New York.

Ylinen, J. Cash, M. 1988. *Sports Massage*. Ebury Press, London.

Zatsiorsky, V.M. 2011. *Biomechanics of Skeletal Muscle*. Human Kinetics, Champaign.

Papers

Akuthota, V. & Chou, L.H. 2004. Sports and performing arts medicine. 2. shoulder and elbow overuse injuries in sports. *Arch. Phys. Med. Rehabil.*, Vol. 85, Suppl. 1, March 2004.

Banks, K. P., et al. 2005. Overuse Injuries of the upper extremity in the competitive athlete: magnetic resonance imaging findings associated with repetitive trauma. *Curr. Probl. Diagn. Radiol.* July/August, 2005.

Barnard, D. 2000. The effect of passive 'soft tissue release' on elbow range of movement and spasticity when applied to the elbow flexors and forearm supinators of a hemiplegic stroke patient – a single case study. Brighton University.

Bell-Jenje, T.C., Gray, J. 2005. Incidence, nature and risk factors in shoulder injuries of national academy cricket players over 5 years – a retrospective study. *SAJSM*, Vol. 17 No. 4.

Blanch, P. 2004. Conservative management of shoulder pain in swimming. *Physical Therapy in Sport*, 5 (2004) pp.109–124.

Cantu, R., Grodin & A.J. DeLany. 1992. Connective tissue perspectives. *J. of Bodywork and Movement Therapies*, 4(4), pp.273–275.

Casale, L. 2001. Physical training for tennis players, *Pdf, S.U.I.S.M.* Torino.

Commerford, M.J. & Mottram, S.L. 2000. Functional stability re-training – principles and strategies for managing mechanical dysfunction. *J. of Manual Therapy*, 6(1), pp.3–14.

Commerford, M.J. & Mottram, S.L. 2000. Movement and stability dysfunction – contemporary developments. *J. of Manual Therapy*, 6(1), pp.15–26.

Cook, T.M. & Farrell, K. 1997. Effects of restricted knee flexion and walking speed on the vertical ground reaction force during gait. *J. of Orthopaedic Sports Physical Therapy*, 25:4, pp.236-244.

Cronin J B, Oliver M, McNairn P J. 2004. Muscle stiffness and injury effects of whole body vibration. *Physical Therapy in Sport*, 5, pp.68–74.

Dennis, R. J. & Finch, C. F. 2008. The reliability of musculoskeletal screening tests used in cricket. *Physical Therapy in Sport*, 9, pp.25–33.

Ebaugh, D.D. & McClure, P.W. 2006. Effects of shoulder muscle fatigue caused by repetitive overhead activities on scapulothoracic and glenohumeral kinematics. *J. of Electromyography and Kinesiology*, 16, pp.224–235.

Eneida, Y.S. et al. 2009. Influence of ankle functional instability on the ankle electromyography during landing after volleyball blocking. *J. of Electromyography and Kinesiology*, 19, pp.84–93.

Feipel, V. & Rondelet, B. 1999. Normal global motion of the cervical spine: an electrogoniometric study. *Clinical Biomechanics*, 14, pp.462–470.

Hase, K. et al. 2002. Biomechanics of rowing. *JSME International*, Vol. 45, No.4.

Hirth, C.J. 2007. Clinical evaluation and testing. *Athletic Therapy Today*.

Holey, E.A. 2000. Connective tissue massage – a bridge between complementary and orthodox approaches. *J. of Bodywork and Movement Therapies*, 4(1), pp.72–80.

Horan, S.A., Evans, K. & Morris, N.R. 2010. Thorax and pelvis kinematics during the downswing of male and female skilled golfers. *Journal of Biomechanics*, 43, pp.1456–1462.

Huard, J., Li, Y. & Fu, F. 2002. Muscle injuries and repair: current trends in research. *The Journal of Bone and Joint Surgery.*

Jebson, P.J.L. & Steyers, C.M. 1997. Hand injuries in rock climbing: reaching the right treatment. *The Physician and Sports Medicine,* Vol. 25, 5, May.

Johnson, J.N., Gauvin, J. & Fredericson, M. 2003. Swimming biomechanics and injury prevention. *The Physician and Sports Medicine,* Vol, 31, 1, January.

Judson, R. 2003, Lawn Bowls Coaching, pdf.

Juhan, D. 1987. In J. DeLany, Connective tissue perspectives. *J. of Bodywork and Movement Therapies*, 4(4), pp.273–275.

Kibler, W B et al. 1996. Shoulder range of motion in elite tennis players: effect of age and years of tournament play. Am. *J. Sports Med.*, 24:279.

Krivkkas, L.S. & Feinberg, J.H. 1996. Lower extremity injuries in college athletes: relation between ligamentous laxity and lower extremity muscle tightness. *Arch. Phyr. Med. Rehab.*, Vol.77, November.

Lichtwarka, G.A. & Wilson, A.M. Optimal muscle fascicle length and tendon stiffness for maximising gastrocnemius efficiency during human walking and running. *J. of Theoretical Biology*, 252, pp.662–673.

Lowe, W.W. 1999. Active engagement strokes. *J. of Bodywork and Movement Therapies*, 4(4), pp.277–278.

Malliaras, P., Cook. J.L. & Kent, P. 2006. Reduced ankle dorsiflexion range may increase the risk of patellar tendon injury among volleyball players. *J. of Science and Medicine in Sport*, (2006) 9, pp.304–309.

Mazzone, T. 1988. Kinesiology of rowing stroke. *NCSA Journal*, Vol.10 No.2.

McGreath, A. & Finch, C. 1996. Bowling cricket injuries over: review of literature. Monash University.

McHardy, A.J. & Pollard, H.P. 2006. A comparison of the modern and classic golf swing: a clinician's perspective. *SAJSM*,18 (3).

McHardy, A.J. & Pollard, H.P. 2007. Golf-related lower back injuries: an epidemiological survey. *Journal of Chiropractic Medicine*, 6, 20–26.

Myers, T.W.1997. The 'anatomy trains', part 2. *J. of Bodywork and Movement Therapies*, 1(3), pp.134–145.

Oschman, J.L. 1997. What is healing energy? Gravity, structure and emotions. *J. of Bodywork and Movement Therapies*, 1(5), pp.297–309.

Oschman, J.L. 1997. In J. DeLany, 'connective tissue perspectives'. *J. of Bodywork and Movement Therapies*, 4(4), pp.273–275.

Pearce, C.J. & Brooks, J.H.M. 2011. The epidemiology of foot injuries in professional rugby union players. *Foot and Ankle Surgery*, 17, pp.113–118.

Peters, P. 2001. Orthopedic problems in sport climbing. *Wilderness and Environmental Medicine*, 12, pp.100–110.

Phadke, V., Camargo, P. R. & Ludewig, P.M. Scapular and rotator cuff muscle activity during arm elevation: a review of normal function and alterations with shoulder impingement. *Rev. Bras. Fisioter.*, 13(1), pp.1-9.

Pluim, B.M., Staal, J.B., Windler, G.E. & Jayanthi ,N. 2006. Tennis injuries: occurrence, aetiology, and prevention. *Br. J. Sports Med.*, 40, pp.415–423.

Rempel, D.M., Keir, P.J. & Bach, J.M. 2008. Effect of wrist posture on carpal tunnel pressure while typing. *J. of Orthopaedic Research*, September.

Stuelckena, M. C., Ginnb, K.A. & Sinclair, P.J. 2008. Shoulder strength and range of motion in elite female cricket fast bowlers with and without a history of shoulder pain. *J. of Science and Medicine in Sport*, 11, pp. 575–580.

Williams, D. 1995. In J. DeLany, Connective tissue perspectives. *J. of Bodywork and Movement Therapies,* 4(4), pp.273–275.

You, J.Y. & Lee, H.M. 2009. Gastrocnemius tightness on joint angle and work of lower extremity during gait. *Clinical Biomechanics*, 24, pp.744–750.

Index

Abdominal muscles, 11
Active STR, 22
Adhesion, 9, 10
Adhesive tissue, 14
Ankle, 153; joints of the, 156; sprains and strains, 168
Antagonists, 11
Archery, 35
Arches, 174
Arthrokinematic movement, 31, 47, 50, 51, 96, 138
Assessment, 13
Atlanto-axial joint, 29, 30
Atlanto-occipital joint, 29, 30
Atrophy, 10, 15
Autonomic responses, 24

Bending over, 106
Blood supply, 15
Body temperature changes, 24
Bone, 10
Bony tunnels, 15
Brachial plexus, 15
Breathing pattern, 23
Brushing hair, 58
Bucket handle, 98

Capillaries, 9
Carpal tunnel, 15
Carrying angle, 75
Cartilage, 10
Cellular debris, 10
Climbing, 90
Closed chain, 119, 139
Collagen, 9, 10
Communication skills, 13
Compartment syndrome, 14
Conditioning, 11
Congested tissue, 11
Connective tissue, 9, 10
Connective tissue (CTM) lock, 18
Contusions, 9
Coupled motion, 31, 32, 96, 100

Cross-bridges, 14
Cycling, 35, 123

Day-to-day activity, 12
Direction of movement, 23
Driving, 35
Dynamic activity, 12

Elbow joint, 73; movement of, 74; range of motion, 74
Endomysium, 7
Epimysium, 7

Fascia, 7, 9, 10, 16
Feel, 13
Feldenkrais method, 11
Fibroblastic activity, 14
Fibroblasts, 9
Fibroplastic activity, 9
Fibula, 15
Foot, joints of the, 156; common problems, 162
Force couples, 52
Forearms, 20, 83

Glenohumeral joint, 45, 50, 51
Golf, 57
Grade of injury, 10
Granular tissue, 10

Hands, 20, 84
Head, 25
High jump, 106
Hip joint, 117; normal ranges for passive movement, 119
Hockey, 106
Hypermobility syndrome, 74
Hypertonic muscle tissue, 14, 16

Iliotibial band friction syndrome, 7
Imbalance, 12
Immobilisation, 10, 11
Inflammation, 9, 14
Inhibited muscles, 11, 14
Intermuscular haematoma, 9

Intramuscular haematoma, 9
Intramuscular nerves, 9

Joints of Luschka, 29, 31

Knee, 137

Lacerations, 9
Lateral epicondylitis, 7, 14
Ligamentous tissue, 9
Ligaments, 7, 10, 16
Lock – lengthen – release, 18
Lumbar spine, lordosis, 100; movements of, 100
Lumbopelvic rhythm, 118
Lumbosacral, motion, 101; spine, 99
Lymphatic tissue, 10

Maintenance, 16
Mandible, movement of the, 27
Manual pressure, 16
Mastication, 26
Median nerve, 15
Microscopic level, 11
Mobility, 9
Motion, ankle joint, 155
Movement, 16; clavicle, 49; elbow, 76; foot through the ankle, 160; gross observational, 47; hip joint, 121; humerus, 55; integrated, 51; knee joint, 143; neck, 33; pattern, 13; restrictions, 7; scapula, 55; selection, 23; shoulder girdle, 48; shoulders, 47; temporomandibular joint, 26; toes, 160; thoracic and lumbosacral spine, 104; wrist and hand, 85, 88
Muscle, 16; ankle and foot, 158; balance, 11; compression, 15; elbow, 76; fibre, 7; forearm, wrist and hand, 87; hip joint, 120; knee joint complex, 18, 142; mass, 10; neck, 32; restrictions, effects of, ankle, 162; restrictions, effects of, elbow, 78; restrictions, effects of, forearm, 90; restrictions, effects of, head and neck, 35; restrictions, effects of, hip, 123; restrictions, effects of, knee, 144; restrictions, effects of, shoulder girdle, 57; restrictions, effects of, temporomandibular

joint, 28; restrictions, effects of, thoracic and lumbosacral, 106; shortening, 15; shoulder, 54; strength, 15; synergies for movement, 52; temporomandibular joint, 27; tissue, 10; tone, 15
Musculotendinous junction, 10
Myofascia, 7, 16

Nausea, 24
Neck, 29
Nerve impulses, 15
Neural tension, 15
Neuromuscular junctions, 9

Open-chain ROM, 119, 138, 156
Osteoarthritis, 117
Osteokinematic movement, 29, 31, 86, 96, 97, 100, 138, 154
Overuse injury, 11, 12; prevention of, 13
Overview, 23

Pain, 7
Palpation, 13; tool, 23
Passive STR, 21
Patellofemoral joint, 141
Perimysium, 7
Periosteum, 7
Peroneal nerve, 15
Physical jobs, 17
Pilates, 11
Piriformis syndrome, 15
Plantar fascia, 157
Postural habits, 12
Pressure, 16, 18
Prevention, 17
Pronation, 156
Proprioception, 11
Proximal tibiofibular joint, 142
Pump action, 98

Q angles, 138

Range of motion (ROM), 10, 13
Recapillarisation, 10
Repair process, 9, 11, 16
Repetitive activity, 12

Resisted STR, 22

Responses (unusual), 24

Rest, ice, compression and elevation (RICE), 14

Restriction, 10

Rib cage motion, 98

Rotation, 26; anterior, 31; clavicular, 51; patella, 141

Rowing, 144

Rugby, 162

Running, 144

Rupture, 9

Sarcomeres, 10

Scapulohumeral rhythm, 51

Scarring, 9–11, 15

Scar tissue, 14, 18

Screw-home mechanism, 141

Shearing, 9

Shoulder, 45; girdle, 45, 46; impingement, 7

Sitting down and picking up objects, 123

Skiing, 123

Soft tissue release to the; adductors in standing, 135; adductors in supine, 133; anconeus in supine, 81; ankle, 163; anterior compartment in supine, 167; biceps brachii and brachialis in supine, 79; brachioradialis in supine, 80; coracobrachialis and biceps brachii (long and short heads) in supine, 71; deep lateral rotators in prone, 131; deep lateral rotators in side lying, 131; deep posterior compartment in prone, 166; deep posterior compartment in side lying, 166; deltoids in seated, 66; deltoids in side lying, 66; deltoid (anterior) in supine, 67; diaphragm in supine, 113; elbow, 79; erector spinae in prone, 107; erector spinae in seated, 109; erector spinae in side lying, 42, 109; finger extensors in supine, 94; finger flexors in supine, 94; foot, 169; foot evertors in supine, 169; foot evertors in side lying, 170; foot invertors in supine, 170; gluteus maximus in prone, 127; gluteus maximus in side lying, 129; gluteus medius and minimus in prone, 129; gluteus medius and minimus and the TFL in side lying, 129; hamstrings and adductor magnus in standing, 135; hamstrings in prone, 149; hamstrings in side lying, 133, 151; hamstrings in supine, 132, 152; hand abductors in supine, 94; hand adductors in supine, 94; head and neck, 36; hip, 124; iliacus in side lying, 125; iliacus in supine, 125; infraspinatus and teres minor in prone, 69; ; intercostals (internal and external) in side lying, 114; intercostals (internal and external) in supine, 114; knee, 145; knee (anterior) in supine, 147; knee in weight bearing, 148; knee (posterior) in prone, 150; knee (posterior) in supine, 151; knee in side lying, 151; lateral compartment in supine, 166; lateral compartment in side lying, 167; latissimus dorsi and teres major in prone, 70; latissimus dorsi and teres major in side lying, 69; levator scapulae in seated, 40, 63; levator scapulae in supine, 40; medial and lateral malleoli in prone, 165; obliques (external and internal) in seated, 112; obliques (external and internal) in supine, 112; pectoralis major in supine, 60; pectoralis minor in supine, 61; plantar fascia in supine, 171; pronator quadratus in supine, 81; pronator teres in supine, 81; psoas major and minor in supine, 124; quadratus lumborum in seated, 111; quadratus lumborum in side lying, 110; quadriceps (and TFL) in seated, 145; quadriceps in side lying – freeing up the ITB, 148; quadriceps in supine, 146; rectus abdominis in seated, 111; rectus abdominis in supine, 111; rectus femoris, sartorius and TFL in side lying, 125; rectus femoris, sartorius and TFL in supine, 127; scalenes (anterior, medius and posterior) in supine, 37; serratus anterior in side lying, 59; serratus anterior in supine, 60; shoulder girdle, 59; spine and thorax, 107; splenius capitis and splenius cervicis in seated, 41; splenius capitis and splenius cervicis in side lying, 41; splenius capitis and splenius cervicis in supine, 40; sternocleidomastoid in supine, 36; subclavius in supine, 62; suboccipitals, 43; superficial compartment in weight bearing, 165; superficial posterior compartment in prone, 163; superficial posterior compartment in side lying, 165; supinator in supine, 81; supraspinatus in prone, 68; supraspinatus in seated, 68; supscapularis in supine, 69; thoracolumbar fascia, 115; thumb abductors in supine, 93; thumb adductors in supine, 93; thumb extensors in supine, 93; thumb flexors in supine, 93; thumb opposition muscles in supine, 93; TMJ in supine, 43; toe abductors in supine, 173; toe adductors in supine, 174; toe extensors in supine, 172; toe flexors in supine, 173; transversospinales in prone, 109; transversospinales in side lying, 110; transversospinales in supine, 42; trapezius in seated, 38; trapezius in supine, 38; trapezius (upper fibres) and levator scapulae in prone, 63; trapezius (upper fibres) and levator scapulae in side lying, 64; trapezius (lower fibres) in prone, 62; trapezius (middle fibres) and rhomboids in prone, 65; trapezius (middle fibres) and rhomboids in seated, 64; trapezius (middle fibres) and rhomboids in side lying, 65; trapezius (upper fibres) in seated, 62; triceps brachii in prone, 80; triceps brachii in supine, 80; triceps brachii (long head) in side lying, 71; wrist abductors in supine, 92; wrist adductors, 92; wrist and hand, 90; wrist extensors in supine, 91; wrist flexors in supine, 91

Soft tissue tunnels, 15
Speed (of application), 23
Sprains, 9
Squash, 90
Static activity, 12
Static positions, 17
Sternoclavicular, 50
Stretch, 21
Supination, 156
Supraspinatus tendonitis, 14
Surface area, 19
Surgery, 15
Surgical repair, 9
Swimming, 58
Synergists, 11

Tarsal tunnel, 15
Tearing, 14
Technique, 18
Temporomandibular joint, 25
Tendinopathy, 11
Tendons, 7, 10, 16, 18
Thoracic spine, 96; movements of, 96; muscles of, 102
Tibial nerve, 15
Tibiofemoral joint, 138
Timing, 24

Tiredness, 24
Tissue congestion, 11
Tissue dysfunction, 12
Tissue release, 11
Tissue tear, 9
Tissue texture, 16
Torso, 95
Training effect, 12
Translation, 26; anterior, 31; distal-proximal, 141; lateral-medial, 141, 156
Treatment of injury, 17
Treatment of layers, 23
Tri-planar motion, 156
Trochoginglymus joint, 74
Typing, 90

Uncinate processes, 29

Versatility, 17
Volleyball, 162

Walking, 144
Wastage (muscle), 11
Weight-bearing STR, 22
Windlass mechanism, 157
Wrist, structure, 84

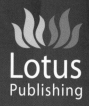

Lotus Publishing

cle Energy Techniques: A Practical Guide for Therapists

Gibbons · 978 1 905367 23 8 · **£19.99**
pages · 275 x 212mm · paperback

practical guide, packed full of colour photographs, illustrates the
ry and practice of muscle energy techniques (MET). The principles
ribed can be incorporated very quickly and effectively into a
ment plan, and can be used to assist in the rehabilitation of anyone
is recovering from an injury.

ial Release for Structural Balance

es Earls and Thomas Myers · 978 1 905367 18 4 · **£24.99**
pages · 275 x 212mm · paperback

al Release for Structural Balance combines manual therapy skills
the exciting new field of structural therapy, which employs the
ue and newly discovered properties of fascial tissues. Through
med assessment and manipulation of fascial patterns, you can help
icate many of your clients' chronic strain patterns—for good.

Tissue Release: A Practical Handbook for Physical Therapists, Third Edition

Mary Sanderson · 978 1 905367 37 5 · **£14.99**
· 168 pages · 275 x 212mm · paperback

Originally written in 1998 as the first book on soft tissue release, this book
has since gone on to sell many 1000s of copies. It has been instrumental
in making soft tissue release a vital tool in the therapist's range of
techniques that can be offered to clients. The book has been updated
and is published in colour for the first time, including new photography
and drawings to illustrate the theory and techniques involved.